Nursing Practice, Policy and Change

Edited by

Marjorie Gott RN, PhD, FRSM

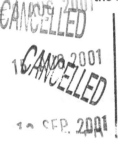
Radcliffe Medical Press

Radcliffe Medical Press
18 Marcham Road, Abingdon, Oxon OX14 1AA

British Library Cataloguing in Publication Data

A catalogue record for this book is available from the British Library.

ISBN 1 85775 351 8

Typeset by Joshua Associates Ltd., Oxford
Printed and bound by TJ International Ltd., Padstow, Cornwall

Contents

Foreword

This book is a brilliant blend of health policy and nursing practice. It identifies the forces that have dominated change in the national health systems of industrialised countries – the shift of priorities from hospital to ambulatory care, the vast expansion in modern technology, the rise in expenditures and efforts at cost-containment, the renewed emphasis on disease prevention and health promotion.

At the same time, this book brings to life the impact of these forces on the actual practice of nursing. It shows through case studies in three major countries ways for nurses to maximise their contribution to patient care and to contribute to the improved effectiveness and efficiency of national health systems.

The demands for medical care have been increasing throughout the world for many reasons: aging of the population, increased education, technological advances, and extended economic support (through insurance and taxation). With this trend the roles of nurses have steadily changed to encompass a broader range of functions. To perform these functions, nursing education is being substantially enriched. The more comprehensively trained nurse is able to take on an independent role, either as nurse practitioner or community health nurse. In these roles, she endows health teams with an orientation toward disease prevention and health promotion.

In the twentieth century, the position of nursing has made many gains in national health systems. It has been strenghtened by advanced education, expansion of clinical practice, appropriate participation in health teams, involvement in decision making or policy, collaboration with other groups to achieve equity in the operation of national health systems. These gains have required hard work and commitment.

In the chapters that follow, nurses from three major countries explore the role of nurse practitioners in evolving national health systems. As these systems change from regarding healthcare as a market commodity to regarding it as a social service, the nurse practitioner has an expanding role to play. She becomes the catalyst in health teams devoted to promoting the well-being of all sectors of human populations.

Marjorie Gott, who is principally responsible for this book, is trained in nursing, with graduate studies in sociology; she is the personal embodiment of health services leadership. She demonstrates in these pages how 'technology' and 'caring' can be harmonised for the most effective operation of national health systems.

Milton I Roemer MD
Professor of Health Services, Emeritus
University of California, Los Angeles
January 2000

Preface

This book is about delivering more and better healthcare, cost effectively. The key to this is better use of the largest sector of the healthcare workforce: nurses.

Nurses are an underused healthcare asset and the purpose of this book is to illustrate their worth and value. Drawing on case studies from the UK, the USA and Australia, authors identify the contributions nurses working at advanced practice level are making to deliver safe, effective and efficient nursing and healthcare to local communities. Using nurses as the first point of contact with the health service is the new direction that healthcare is beginning to take worldwide, as health policy makers seek better value for the 'healthcare dollar' by reorienting service provision away from 'after the event' hospital care, towards (prevention-led) primary healthcare.

Working in a range of settings, from inner city areas to remote communities, the nurses described in this book demonstrate that they can make a difference to healthcare. Across a range of services they deliver care that is at least equal to that provided by other healthcare workers (principally doctors), and, in some cases, better. Nurses are flexible, multi-skilled, good value, well accepted and are keen to develop new skills and advance their education. They demand more policy attention and investment than they received in the previous century. Investment in higher education for nurses appears to offer a particularly good return. In the UK, the USA and Australia, educated nurse practitioners are frequently to be found leading the way in innovative, entrepreneurial, community-responsive good practice.

Marjorie Gott
January 2000

List of contributors

UK

Margaret Bamford RN, PhD, MSc is Chairman of Dudley Priority NHS Trust.

Naomi Chambers BA, DipHSM, PhD is Senior Fellow at the Health Services Management Unit, University of Manchester and Non-Executive member of Southern Derbyshire Health Authority.

Marjorie Gott RN, PhD, FRSM is Director of Gott Associates, International Health Service Research and Education Consultants.

USA

Kara M Connors MPH is the Associate Director of Community–Campus Partnerships for Health, and was the Program Coordinator for the Health Professions Schools in Service to the Nation Program (1995–1998).

Rosemary Goodyear RN, FNP, EDD is Visiting Professor at the School of Nursing, University of South Florida.

Joanne Kirk Henry EdD, RNCS is Director of the Community Nursing Organization, Associate Professor at Virginia Commonwealth University, and was the Director of the Health Professions Schools in Service to the Nation Program (1995–1998).

Sarena D Seifer MD is the Executive Director of Community–Campus Partnerships for Health, and was the Program Director for the Health Professions Schools in Service to the Nation Program (1995–1998).

Australia

Sally Borbasi RN, MA, PhD is Senior Lecturer in Nursing at Adelaide University.

Judi Brown RN, DipEd, MEd is Principal Project Officer, Statewide Services Division, Department of Human Services, Government of South Australia.

Pauline Donnelly RHV, BNurs, MHM is Commonwealth Nursing Officer, Commonwealth of Australia Department of Health and Aged Care, Adelaide, Australia.

Denise Hegney RN, PhD, FRCNA is Professor of Rural Nursing, University of Southern Queensland, Toowoomba, Queensland, Australia.

Alan Pearson RN, PhD, FRCNA is Professor of Nursing at La Trobe University, Melbourne.

David White RN, BSc, MEd is Chief Nursing Officer, Statewide Services Division, Department of Human Services, Government of South Australia.

List of abbreviations

AIHW	Australian Institute of Health and Welfare
AMA	American Medical Association
ANA	American Nurses Association
APN	Advanced Practice Nurse
CCPH	Community–Campus Partnerships for Health
CE	Continuing Education
CPHVA	Community Practitioners and Health Visitors Association
DN	Doctoral Nursing
ENB	English National Board for Nursing, Midwifery and Health Visiting
EPSDT	Early Periodic Screening and Development Testing (Program)
EU	European Union
FNP	Family Nurse Practitioner
GP	General Practitioner
HD	Health Department
HFA	Health for All
HMO	Health Maintenance Organisation
HPSISN	Health Professions Schools in Service to the Nation (Program)
HRSA	Department of Health Resources and Service Administration
HSC	Health Science Center
MCO	Managed Care Organisations
NAMIPPA	Nurses and Midwives in Private Practice, Australia
NGT	Nominal Group Techique
NHS	National Health Service
NHSE	National Health Service Executive
NLMIS	Nurse-Led Minor Injuries Service
NLMIU	Nurse-Led Minor Injuries Unit
NONPF	National Organisation of Nurse Practitioner Faculties
NP	Nurse Practitioner
NUPRAC	Nurse Practitioner (Project)
OECD	Organisation for Economic Co-operation and Development
PAGC	Prince Albert Grand Council
PCG	Primary Care Group
PCP	Primary Care Provider
PFI	Private Finance Initiative
PHC	Primary Healthcare
PHD	Public Health Departments
PHN	Public Health Nurse/Nursing
PREP	Post-Registration Education and Practice
RAN	Remote Area Nurse

RCN	Royal College of Nursing
RFDS	Royal Flying Doctor Service
SON	School of Nursing
UKCC	United Kingdom Central Council for Nurses, Midwives and Health Visitors
WHO	World Health Organisation
WIC	Women, Infants and Children (Program)

Seeing nursing

CHAPTER ONE

Nursing practice, policy and change

Marjorie Gott

> *Because of their in-depth knowledge and experience, they have much to offer in the areas of healthcare assessment and policy development.*
> (1996 World Health Organisation Expert Committee)

Good things are said about nurses. They are showered with praise and exhalted in rhetoric. Yet conversations with nurses around the world, at the turn of the century, indicate a profession in crisis. Despite the large gains that nursing has made during the 20th century, in practice, in education and in research, there remain misgivings and anxieties about the future. This book explores some of the reasons for these anxieties and offers some positive ways forward.

Conversations with senior nurses in Britain, Australia and America revealed that nurses working on the three continents share similar challenges. These provide a focus for this book.

Although the systems in which they work differ, these nurses were unanimous in their plea for nursing to finally realise its potential as a shaper of health service policy rather than (in spite of its size) a 'bit-part' player. They were also unanimous in urging authors to look forward rather than backwards and concentrate on finding and describing the case studies of good nursing practice. Doing this necessitates choosing case studies for analysis. Although a degree of serendipity was inevitably involved, the case studies chosen were influenced by awareness of trends and recurrent themes arising from discussions. More is said about this in the next chapter. Firstly, it is necessary to review our position as nurses at the turn of the century.

Influences on nursing

The previous three decades in particular have seen major changes in healthcare thinking and provision. Change offers opportunities as well as limitations, but generally nurses have not been prepared to recognise and exploit change. This may be due to their professional insecurity. Fulton (1997) alleges that:

> *Nurses suffer lack of confidence and self esteem and represent themselves as an oppressed group.*

To understand why this is so it is necessary to identify and explore significant influences on nursing in the 20th century. Foremost amongst these have been medicine, gender and technology. Their influences have been interconnected.

Medicine

Other health service colleagues help set the health service, and thus nursing's, education and practice agenda. The dominance of one particular professional group, physicians, throughout the 20th century, has skewed healthcare thinking and healthcare work in a particular direction (scientific medicine); this has delayed and prejudiced the development of nursing as a discipline.

In addition to laying down scientific medicine (the medical model) as the only valid way to think about and plan healthcare services, the medical profession formed a unique and powerful alliance with governments to protect their interests. Whilst health services in the western world were subject to frequent and wide-ranging changes during the 20th century, the one thing that changed very little was the power relationship between doctors and governments. Talking about how this relationship has affected nursing in the United Kingdom (UK) Salter (1998) alleges:

> *Nursing exists within a state-sponsored system of medical hegemony . . . Nursing's traditional role in the politics of change in the NHS was to provide the appropriate support to the concordat between medicine and the state.*

Reflecting on the bids for autonomy that nursing has made in the last decades of the 20th century, Salter is pessimistic. He alleges that by distancing themselves from medicine nurses have lost their power base. That is an argument that this book acknowledges but does not concede.

The inter-professional rivalries and turf wars that characterised 20th century healthcare were in nobody's long-term interest, and certainly not the patients that the system is meant to serve. The current world-wide reorientation of healthcare, with its emphasis on collaborative development of good practice, demands both that health professionals work together more effectively, and that governments more rigorously address the value they are getting for the healthcare dollar, and who best can deliver it. Traditional views, roles and practises will change as these issues are addressed.

Gender

As a predominately female profession practising in a male-delineated world order nursing was relatively powerless for much of the century. In the late 1960s and during the 1970s, however, the anti-conservative liberation movements that swept the developed world, with their emphasis on reducing oppression (gender, race, 'big' business interests) brought feminine interests and values to the fore. Feminine values are holistic and inclusive, rather than individual and exclusive (male). They offer the potential for a different kind of healthcare that focuses on the long- rather than the short-term, and the broad, rather than the narrow gaze. Thinking about the social future, Giddens (1996) urges incorporation of the female perspective into welfare planning.

Internationally, the health policy script is being rewritten and women are stepping into the spotlight. But in the future will they play a minor or a major role? This is a crucially important question that will concern nursing as it seeks to progress.

The influence of emancipatory politics can be seen in the radical ideological shift in its relationship with medicine that nursing made in the 1970s. Up until then nursing policy had been largely bound up with, and frequently dependent upon, medical policy. In the last third of the century nurses challenged and changed the nature of their relationship with medical theory and practice and embraced a social, as opposed to a medical, model of health.

The social model of health is concerned with the conditions and contexts that shape health opportunities and experiences. Inevitably these are connected with susceptibilities towards illness and disease (the medical model of 'health', in which health is defined as absence of disease). The social model of health encompasses the medical model, rather than standing as an alternative account of health opportunities and illness experiences. Recognition of the value of the social model of health has been responsible for the development of the health promotion paradigm. Health promotion has three main branches of activity:

- preventive care, involving screening for early signs of disease; immunisation to prevent disease occurring
- health education, involving both individual 'risk reduction' advice and broader community-wide campaigns (such as the long-running 'Look After Your Heart' campaigns in the UK, USA and Australia)
- health protection, involving remedial and rehabilitative care, and also measures concerned with improving living and working contexts, often through legislation (healthy schools and workplaces).

Health promotion work is an expansion of their role that nurses are increasingly embracing, both as a branch of practice and as an extension to their existing clinical work.

Technology

Like medicine, technology has, until recently, been a predominantly male concern. Knowledge about and use of information technology is a fundamental tool of enfranchisement in the 20th century. The concern for nurses is that women have been slow to embrace the information society, and when they have the evidence is that the gender segregation that affected women in traditional work is being repeated; men design the projects; women punch in the data (Houdart-Blazy, 1996).

As women and female practitioners, nurses may be doubly disadvantaged. But the signs are that this is now being recognised and addressed with programmes to bring women into technology. In Europe, a Year for Women (Houdart-Blazy, 1996) had technological literacy as its core project and European Union-funded projects were redirected towards multidisciplinary project design and realisation. Female values were celebrated as bringing a more multifaceted and holistic (and therefore client friendly) approach to project design, and creativity was encouraged.

Use of the information society is both the main challenge and opportunity facing women today. The potential exists for nurses to initiate, develop and showcase change in practice.

A European Union-funded project (Gott, 1995) explored the use of accessible, low-cost social technologies (telephone, television etc.) to promote the health and well-being of society. Tele (at a distance) health was contrasted with the main (and most expensive) form of telematic research in healthcare: telemedicine. Telemedicine is principally concerned with 'after the event' illness care rather than (preventing the event) health promotion. Case studies of good practice, led by nurses and others, make the case for reorientation of health policy away from an obsession with costly (and frequently dubious) high-tech 'solutions' towards lower cost, more socially inclusive forms of health and illness promotion and protection.

> . . . *Looking back urges us to be cautious about 'progress'.
> Reviewing Western healthcare this century, the inescapable
> conclusion is that the major growth area ('after the event'
> service provision) got in the way of society's real need: health
> protection and promotion.*   (Gott, 1995)

Nursing practice and health policy

In the 1980s, advances in nursing curricula and relocation into the higher education sector led to increased weighting in the behavioural, as opposed to the biological, sciences as part of the curriculum, increasing reliance on social models and accounts of health. These changes allowed for further advances in nursing practice and further development of the clinical expert nurse role. The predominant health-care trend in the 1980s was one in which, worldwide, governments in developed societies were starting to address the 'pay off' investing in disease (secondary care) had yielded, and were switching resources to primary care. This brought new opportunities for advanced nursing practice.

The 1990s has seen increasing policy commitment to (within budget) reorientation of healthcare towards care in the community. This is cost driven in the face of massive and rising health and welfare costs. A new model of health, the commodities model, has been adopted. This model is neither medical nor social, but economic. It is similar, however, to the medical model in that it is reductionist in vision and fragmentary in practice. Budgets are allocated and targets are set in relation to specific diseases and activities; the focus is the individual rather than the community. This poses a new dilemma for nurses.

Nursing practice is limited by the context and conditions in which it takes place. Health service work is big business and, although nurses are the largest sector of the healthcare workforce, they are not the most influential. Governments decide health policy, nurses enact it. This can cause a conflict of interest for nurses when inherent professional beliefs and values are challenged by restrictions in their practice necessary to meet externally imposed (government) health targets.

Gott and O'Brien (1990) studied the role of the nurse in health promotion and found that nurses' roles and relationships are proscribed by both the structural and ideological contexts that nurses find themselves in. There was evidence of conflicting agenda being set for a major and growing aspect of the nurse's role; health promotion with individuals and communities. This led to role conflict for practitioners. This situation was compounded by the low (political) status in which nursing is generally held, which limits nurses' ability to participate fully in effecting structural changes for health.

They found that, although educated differently, in practice, when doing health promotion work, nurses adopted an individualistic focus. It is believed they did this because emphasis on individual habits and behaviours is less politically charged than emphasis on the conditions and contexts that shape health and illness experiences. Gott and O'Brien argue that by focusing on the education and risk reduction behaviours of individual citizens, nurses may be acting as agents of social control rather than as agents for social change. They therefore collude in victim-blaming practices and this causes a high degree of anxiety and role dissonance (Gott and O'Brien, 1990):

> *Whilst constituting the largest single body of healthcare workers, the nursing profession is subjected to a series of interprofessional and social pressures which structure the relationships with its client populations. Responding to this system of pressure nurses attempted to situate the 'whole person' as the basis of their practice. Yet in reality, that practice has precisely the opposite effect: it divides people up into categories of behavioural and physiological 'symptoms' which nursing practice can attack. This attack is waged through the twin weapons of personal relationships and information systems. Yet rather than generating control over the determinants of health, the practice divests individuals of their own skills, knowledge and agenda and buries these under risk-factor management programmes.*

Enfranchisement of previously low-power groups (women, nurses) has been referred to earlier. Growing public participation in the democratic process in western societies means that governments need to take account of public concerns and seek to work *with* people rather than *at* them. If governments are to realise their policy objectives they will also need to recognise and validate the concerns of workers in the system, and address the values that they hold. Nursing values are already congruent with the changed direction for healthcare policy; primary healthcare. Switching efforts and resources from secondary (hospital) to primary (community-based) care is now the main policy direction of all western governments. Governments need to recognise that nurses are uniquely placed and prepared to help them in their efforts.

There are now also signs of a more reflective approach to social policy. A backlash against globalisation is growing as people experience ethical concerns about business at any cost, and feelings of power-lessness to limit the free-market hegemony. Leading thinkers (de Alcantara, 1996) are now calling for reappraisal of the direction in which societies are headed, and making a plea for a return to (female, nursing) human scale and human values.

> *The particular form of 'globalisation' currently shaping our lives – with its over-riding emphasis on competition and its degrading lack of concern with human security – is not immutable. It is the product of adherence to an ideology that interprets life as a vicious struggle to be won by the strongest. Such a world view requires modification. Human beings are motivated by solidarity and hope, as well as by selfishness and fear.*

It seems that the ideological tide might be turning in nurses' favour. But they are not quite ready to capitalise on it. Internationally and nationally, professional nursing organisations are exhorting nurses to do things they may not be able to do, at least not without new alliances, partners and skills. Taking the World Health Organisation's lead, professional bodies throughout the developed world have exhorted nurses, during the last decade, to show leadership skills, yet too often have failed to recognise that leadership involves teamwork, negotiation and other management of change skills. Generally, nurses are poorly prepared in these skills. This has now been recognised by WHO (1996a) who comment that nursing includes managing situations that are rapidly changing. In referring to public health nursing, the WHO expert committee on nursing practice notes:

> *Because of their in-depth knowledge and experience, they have much to offer in the areas of healthcare assessment and policy development.*

They go on to note, however, that few health professionals (including nurses) receive management training as part of their professional education. Advanced practice demands these and other skills, in par-ticular management of change and collaborative working.

Because of these deficits, and nursing education's failure to address them, practising nurses continue to experience guilt, confusion and anxiety because they cannot live up to others (and their own, internalised) ideals. This limits both clear thinking and practice development.

In their academic courses of preparation for practice, nurses are educated to see 'the big (healthcare) picture', and, by implication, believe that they can influence it when they begin working as practitioners. In practice their scope has become limited by:

- a lack of a coherent identity
- demoralisation due to working to meet top-down requirements (when they are educated to look for 'bottom-up' ones)
- containment and shrinkage of their role as they become employed and used in different ways [health visitors employed by general practitioners (GPs) in the UK, public health nurses employed by Health Maintenance Organisations (HMOs) in the US].

In order to move forward and realise their potential, nurses need to be aware of the aforementioned historical and social forces that have shaped the conditions and contexts in which they practice. They also need to be aware of how concepts of healthcare are shaped and used by others, as well as themselves. The term 'primary healthcare' has been particularly contentious.

Nurses and primary healthcare

It is now commonly accepted that, in the past, when we spoke of primary healthcare, we largely meant primary medical care (preventive, diagnostic, rehabilitative work). The WHO 'Health For All' movement (WHO, 1978) changed thinking on this, however, by recognising and celebrating public health and placing it centre stage. The worldwide rise of the 'new public health' in the 1970s was readily accepted and well understood by nurses, but when they tried to practice it they found that incongruities existed between their understanding and that of others.

This is because there is a distinction between primary healthcare (PHC) and public health: PHC is much a narrower concept and set of activities than public health. For example, in the UK, GPs have been slow to recognise the need for inter-sectoral collaboration and public participation in health-related decision making, and their focus remains primarily (after the event) disease orientated. UK community nurses, however, have taken a broader view of PHC, encompassing health promotion, as well as disease prevention. Peckham and Macdonald

(1996) allege that such activity is despite the PHC team rather than because of it:

> *many community nurses describe this activity as marginal and often find it hard to gain organisational support from within the practice or from health purchasers.*

They believe community nurses are hampered in their efforts by both 'short-termism' (projects not funded long enough to demonstrate results) and an inability to work inter-sectorally because of the disease hegemony pervading PHC work.

Health managers make health policy, but the key actors influencing health policy decision making have been doctors. Their hegemony can largely be explained in relation to the context in which 'health' care has been practised for most of this century; hospitals. As indicated earlier, however, spiralling health costs and demographic changes have forced health policy makers to reassess the prevent/cure/care balance of health provision and led them to reorient more healthcare spending and activity towards community/primary healthcare. This shift in emphasis in health policy making has occurred throughout the developed world and is changing medical practice and health policy, allowing more and different actors to take a leading role. There are new opportunities for public health nurses to develop and expand the contribution that they can make to improving public health.

It also seems that nurses want to practise a broader notion of PHC than their medical colleagues. At first sight this seems unremarkable, doctors are, after all, trained to deal with illness and disease. Yet the irony is that worldwide (to varying degrees) doctors are being both exhorted and required to do more illness prevention and health promotion work (Department of Health, 1997; Joseph *et al.*, 1997).

This is not what they want to do. For a number of reasons, mainly connected with short-termism, many doctors remain deeply sceptical about the value of health promotion work. Bradley and McKnight (1997) encapsulate their views when discussing postgraduate medical education needs (as voiced by doctors themselves):

> *The least well-attended category was health promotion. While GPs suggested a number of topics which they felt should be the subject of further meetings, many of them reported scepticism about the effectiveness of health promotion strategies and would require more information on the effectiveness of health promotion and various patient interventions.*

Of course it is likely that at least some of these doctors may be sceptical about the way that health promotion targets and strategies may be naïvely (or cynically?) set by government health ministers, who themselves sometimes appear ignorant of the broader concept of public health. The tension is, however, that if public health and quality of life is to improve (and no one wants it to worsen!), someone needs to develop and practice expert health promotion with and for the communities they serve. Nurses working in community and PHC settings have the skills, abilities and aptitudes to do effective and efficient health promotion work. If they can work collaboratively with general practitioners and thus share the strong power base that they exert, they could be a major force for change. Up until now, however, nurses have had limited opportunities and negligent support. It is not surprising therefore that they undervalue themselves and often seem demoralised.

Nursing, as a profession, needs to confront and work through its insecurity. Nurses need to develop the skills necessary to both manage change more effectively and to better market their skills and abilities. They need to become sure about who and what they are and to convince others (particularly health service commissioners) of their worth. The following examples illustrate this.

In the UK, public health nursing is performed by specially trained health visitors. The profession of health visiting has been undergoing a severe identity crisis for a number of years, largely as a result of its failure to adapt to and predict changes occurring in healthcare, and also its inability to convince key health service decision makers of the profession's (quite considerable) potential worth. Because health visiting as a profession has not only failed to move with the times, but, crucially, failed to predict changing social trends and policies, they are seen as a superfluous service by some health service commissioners and numbers employed are falling. Rather late in the day this has prompted a marketing exercise by the Community Practitioners and Health Visitors Association (CPHVA) who issued a position statement (1997) entitled: 'Public Health: the Role of Nurses and Health Visitors.' In the statement they pose the question:' *Why a position statement about public health?*' They go on to acknowledge that:

> *The emphasis on public health in current government policy is welcome, but funding decisions sometimes overlook or misunderstand the importance of school nurses and health visitors in implementing this new agenda.*

More recently (UKCC, 1999), the view was that there were:

> *relatively few published examples of health visitors extend-*
> *ing their practice, unlike the extensive documentation of*
> *such developments in nursing.*

Insecurity about this public health nurse type role was not limited to the UK. The comments of a United States academic were more extreme:

> *Public health nurses are a shrinking work force. Fewer and*
> *fewer are being employed by the Health Departments. But*
> *you know . . . (long pause) I wouldn't have said this a year ago*
> *I sometimes wonder if they've run their course . . . whether*
> *we need public health nurses any more. Many of the things*
> *they do could be done by other workers; health educators or*
> *social workers for example. Do they need to be nurses? . . .*
> *(pause) I'm not sure anymore. (long pause) It's almost as if we*
> *need two types. One to do the individual and family work;*
> *which still needs to be done . . . and the other to do the*
> *community development stuff (pause) I'm not sure.*

Another educator (UK) talked about a recent discussion she had held with her students about the need for a nursing registration prior to taking the health visiting course:

> *They say: 'Oh well, knowledge of disease systems, things like*
> *this, it helps you explain things to people . . .'*

> (She goes on to comment) *. . . but I don't know that that's a*
> *good enough reason . . .I just think it would help them decide*
> *their public health role more effectively if the nursing thing*
> *didn't get in the way.*

A way forward

So there is confusion about public health nursing both in practice and in preparation for practice. Ironically this confusion is surfacing and distracting the profession at a time of great opportunity for community nursing. The worldwide shift to primary healthcare (care in the community), the projected demographic increase in the care burden and the fact that the majority of the care force are nurses offers great opportunities for innovative development of advanced nursing practice. Additionally, at this time, developed countries are seeking to adopt health structures and policies that will use available resources more effect-ively and efficiently. They are also seeking to share the burden of responsibility for health by encouraging people to adopt behaviours that reduce illness incidents and promote health. Nursing personnel form the largest part of the healthcare workforce. Nurses have the opportunity to affect the changing profile, politics and priorities of world health. Slowly, policy makers are realising this. In 1997 the Director General of the World Health Organisation in a speech to the Global Advisory Group on Nursing and Midwifery (WHO, 1997) recognised nurses' potential and called for skills for the 21st century including:

- evidence-based practice
- collaboration with other health professionals with a team-centred and patient-focused approach.

In his view, education in nursing should be as much about learning management skills as it is about gaining clinical knowledge. He says:

> There is an urgent need for nurses to understand reform mechanisms for efficiency, effectiveness and cost contain-ment and to link these directly with health gain and quality of life for their clients and patients.

In his view nurses are clearly seen as a way of improving the economic effectiveness and efficiency of health services. This is in line with economic advice given by the Organisation for Economic Co-operation and Development (OECD, 1994);

> Governments are examining their social programmes, not only to alter any unintended effects, but also to use available resources more prudently . . .Social policy has an obligation to ensure that resources are mobilised more efficiently and effectively . . . for the credibility of the policies themselves as investments in society.

Some practitioners have recognised this and are currently developing visionary projects, often in alliance with other health professionals (Harrison and Neve, 1996; HRSA, 1996). The nursing profession itself, however, and the statutory bodies that govern education and training seem unaware that the world is changing but persist in inward-looking professional institutionalism that separates nurse from nurse and hinders, rather than progresses, the profession.

In the meantime, while this professional soul searching is going on, groups of nurses are moving and growing quickly into new roles, with different and varying forms of preparation and spheres of practice (for example health centre-based practice nurses and managers). In one instance, nurse practitioners, this advanced nurses' role is extending into new work areas and embracing that of other health professionals, most frequently physicians, particularly in the USA.

Nurse practitioners are trained nurses with advanced post-basic education who assume responsibility for health assessment and the management and delivery of services at the first level of a healthcare system. They are a rapidly growing group of advanced nursing practitioners. Their progress is being keenly watched by a number of interested parties, not least governments committed to improving effectiveness and efficiency in health and welfare services.

In the UK, management consultants Touche Ross were requested by the government to review 20 programmes in which nurse practitioners were employed in general practice (physician office) settings. Their conclusions (1994) were that:

- patients were highly satisfied with care given by nurse practitioners
- patients value the broader focus of consultations, including promotion of well-being as well as illness prevention
- there is great scope for the development of the nurse practitioner role in primary healthcare, through jointly managing caseloads with physicians.

Rather than celebrating this new role for nurses, the profession itself seems at best ambivalent and at worst hostile. Nurse practitioners in the US are frequently accused of becoming mini-physicians because of the way their role has developed. They are increasingly being hired by HMOs because they are cheaper than (but as good as) physicians for doing preventative work. But are these nurses selling out or buying in?

Nursing exists to serve the public. This fact sometimes becomes obscured in internal professional debates about 'advancement' of the profession of nursing. When participating in these debates, nurses need to start from the recognition that they belong to a health system. A worldwide authority on health systems (Roemer, 1990) has identified influences on health systems as including:

> *(1) human needs; (2) expanded technology and specialisation; (3) greater health expenditures by society as a whole; (4) expectation of quality performance and (5) achievement of an equitable distribution of health services, according to the diversity of human needs.*

Roemer (1990) identifies a need for greater numbers of skilled health workers, including nurses, to meet current and future health system needs and cites better continuing education and teamworking as vital for the delivery of a safe, efficient and cost-effective health service:

> Doctors who work in teams with nurses, psychologists, dieticians, technicians and others are much more productive at less cost per unit of service. They can provide higher quality services at lower costs.

It could be argued that as long as there is a public need and as long as nurses are adequately trained and have chosen this clinical role as a considered option for professional practice, their practice should be supported and developed. There is a need for clinical work and primary prevention work with high-risk groups in the population, so why shouldn't nurses do it? They have good 'people' and teaching skills and a broader conception of health promotion and disease prevention than that generally held by their colleagues.

A less trivial challenge that might be made against nurse practitioner practice is that their deployment and currently perceived remit will diminish the community-based public health nursing function. This is a serious challenge that needs to be acknowledged, but the debate should not be hedged by interprofessional sniping and rivalry. Shooting the messenger (of change) is not the way forward, better to celebrate and learn from professional diversity. The world of healthcare is changing rapidly; nursing needs to decide whether it wants to lead or follow, and plan accordingly.

Advancing knowledge and practice requires nursing to become more sensitive to and more skilled at dealing with other actors, contexts and interests in the health field. Nurses need to decide what kind of change agent they wish to be: reactive or proactive; do they wish to set agendas for health, or respond to agendas set by others? Inevitably, given different sets of circumstances, societal need and team skills and opportunities, change will be both reactive and proactive. But it could be more proactive than it is. Articulate, informed nurses need to be involved in all levels of health service decision making. Part of their role will be to educate other health service decision makers about the value of nursing and the contribution nursing can make to the health and well-being of society. They can do this by showcasing good nursing and healthcare practice.

'Real-life' best practice, documented, disseminated and extended is increasingly seen as the basis for healthcare decision making and planning worldwide. In 1996 WHO recommended the review, analysis and comparison of successful and innovative experiences from health-care systems (WHO, 1996b). In some developed countries (Northern Europe, the US, Canada and Australia) extensive databases of good nursing practice already exist. The Canadian initiative, a collaborative project between The Canadian Nurses Association and the School of Nursing at McMaster University, aims to disseminate and utilise (nursing) research findings for use by nurses in practice and policy development (Shestowsky, 1997). The Joanna Briggs Institute at the University of Adelaide also does this (http://www.joannabriggs.edu.au), as does the Hardin directory at the University of Iowa (www.lib.uiowa.edu/hardin/md/nurs.html) and the Centre for Evidence-Based Nursing at the University of York (www.york.ac.uk/depts/hstd/centres/evidence/ev-intro.htm).

So the trend that is evolving means that, in the future, advancing nursing education and practice will increasingly rely on building and demonstrating case studies of good practice. This exercise is likely to be a collaborative one and one in which nurses are true (healthcare) team players – not just followers, but leaders. The notion and practice of leadership is changing, however, and deserves some attention here.

The 1980s and 1990s have seen a plethora of publications about leadership and teamworking. The field of primary healthcare in particular has been deluged with re-educative advice, mostly concerned with interdisciplinary working.

The concept of interdisciplinary care is based on the premise that healthcare is delivered by a team, each member having their own set of professional skills. The job of the team leader is to co-ordinate skills to maximise effective and efficient healthcare delivery (yet protectionist working practices may sometimes militate against this). Interdisciplinary care recognises and utilises the different skills of team members, but the margins of care and responsibility are blurred and shared. Leaders are more likely to work jointly and collaboratively to commonly agreed protocols of good practice. Depending upon the issue and the context, protocols are as likely to be initially devised by nurses as by doctors or other teamworkers.

This new form of leadership, and the potential it affords nursing has been recognised by Malby (1997), who summarises the current position very well. She recognises that there is an unrealised potential of skilled therapeutic nursing practice in a changing demography and society and calls for:

> leadership that moves out of the 'expert' mode into a more collaborative and dynamic relationship with an increasingly complex system. Leadership will hinge on relationship building, being willing to create dialogue, and on engaging with all those who have an interest in health services within a local focus. Values will describe the parameters for initiatives and

strategy, and effective and human service delivery will be dependent on information and decision-making being as close to the patient as possible.

Much health-funded research, in Europe in particular, is now orientated towards finding, analysing, disseminating, replicating and building on case studies of good practice in primary healthcare. The emphasis now is very much a grass roots approach: what works, where, why and with whom? Also, where else would it work, and what does it cost?

The author has been involved in a number of European Union research projects over the last two decades. During that time a very definite change has taken place. Whereas formerly large, expensive single-issue projects would receive long-term funding quite easily, now the emphasis is very much on funding small-scale clusters of related projects with shorter stage interim accountability. Families and generations of projects then grow in a more related, useful and accountable fashion.

The European Union (EU) *Tipping The Balance Towards Primary Health Care* Project (Rathwell *et al.*, 1995) was charged with building and reporting case studies of good practice in PHC that showed a true public health orientation by incorporating World Health Organisation 'Health For All' (HFA) principles. A project in Alvsborg County (Sweden) was designed to strengthen confidence in PHC by changing the communication interface between PHC, the hospital and patients. The goal was that people should experience PHC and the hospital as one healthcare organisation, without encountering boundary difficulties. PHC nurses and hospital emergency nurses were trained, using the same specially designed programme, to be responsible for information and telephone counselling communications with the public. The result was that the number of visits to health centres increased, and the number of visits to hospital decreased accordingly. This work has demonstrated the value of re-orientating roles and activities in PHC work and shown that using specially trained nurses as the first point of contact in a PHC encounter is both effective and efficient. Concepts and practices developed in the project have now spread to other sites in Europe.

So current and building evidence is that when nurses do work in an interdisciplinary way they are very good at it. In both the EU *Tipping the Balance* and the EU *Telematics for Health* (Gott, 1995) research projects the following was found:

- in Spain specially trained midwives were found to give as good care and be better accepted than public health doctors
- in Sweden PHC services were reorganised; nurses are the first and only point of contact for many

- in Ireland community mothers, supported by public health nurses, model and teach child-rearing in deprived areas
- in the UK (nurse initiated) neighbourhood forums give local citizens a voice in health service decision making
- in Wales 'at risk' pregnant women manage and monitor pregnancies at home with midwife and obstetrician support.

These case studies of good practice form part of the growing body of evidence that demonstrates nurses' ability to advance both nursing and health service practice.

Before moving on from the issue there is another important point to make here, and it is to do with advocacy. In interdisciplinary work it is invariably the nurse who is the patients' 'champion'. Health settings may differ, but where joint care (shared management protocols), joint planning (locality policy making) and joint research (case studies of good practice) are occurring it is the nurse who brings in the community and its representatives. She has the big picture and it is based on a social model of health (into which the medical/illness model is incorporated). She is pragmatic in terms of what the issues are and how they might be addressed, and, because of her *Health for All* orientation, she is more in tune with societies' needs and capabilities.

Conclusions

As they succeed, nurses will become more secure in their identity and worth, will be understood more and work more effectively with colleagues and be able to do what it is they do best; care for and advance the interests of citizens and communities. The essence of nursing is caring and that can occur at individual, group and societal level – caring enough to make a difference to the quality of life of an individual, group or community. But as a profession we really need to decide where we are going, why and in whose interests. The 20th century was notable for turf wars with each other and with other health professionals. It is now time to look forward and look at what we are good at, accept and celebrate it and get out there and demonstrate it in multiple settings with multiple ranges of skills and practices.

Nurses need to believe in themselves and to believe in the future. They need to be visionaries, able to predict, celebrate and manage change with open and democratic minds. The case studies that are presented in this book show us how this might be done.

References

Bradley T and McKnight A (1997) The education needs of GPs for health promotion in primary care. *International Journal of Health Education* **35** (4): 126–7.

CPHVA (1997) *Public Health: The Role of Nurses and Health Visitors. Position Paper.* Community Practitioners' and Health Visitors' Association, London.

de Alcantara CH (1996) Introduction. *Social Futures, Global Visions.* Blackwell Publishers, Oxford.

Department of Health (1997) *England: The New NHS.* White Paper, Cmnd No 3807. Department of Health, London.

Fulton S (1997) Nurses' views on empowerment: a critical social theory perspective. *Journal of Advanced Nursing* **26**: 529–36.

Giddens A (1996) Affluence, poverty and the idea of a post scarcity society. In: de Alcantara (ed) *Social Futures, Global Visions.* Blackwell Publishers, Oxford.

Gott M (1995) *Telematics for Health. The Role of Telehealth and Telemedicine in Homes and Communities.* Radcliffe Medical Press, Oxford.

Gott M and O'Brien M (1990) *The Role of the Nurse in Health Promotion: Policies, Perspectives and Practices.* Department of Health, London.

Harrison L and Neve H (1996) *A Review of Innovations in Primary Healthcare.* The Policy Press, Bristol.

Houdart-Blazy (1996) *Introduction: The Information Society. . . A Challenge for Women.* Women of Europe Dossier, Issue No 44, European Commission, Brussels.

HRSA (1996) *Models That Work. A Compendium of Innovative Primary Health Care Programs for Underserved and Vulnerable Populations.* United States Department of Health and Human Services, Health Resources and Services Administration, Washington.

Joseph *et al.* (1997) Australia's co-ordinated care trials. *Changing Medical Education and Practice* **Dec**: 10, 11.

Malby R (1997) Developing the future leaders of nursing in the UK. *European Nurse* **2**(1): 27–35.

OECD (1994) Position Paper No 55. Organisation for Economic Co-operation and Development, Geneva.

Peckham S and Macdonald J (1996) *Towards a Public Health Model of Primary Care* (Report). The Public Health Alliance, Birmingham.

Rathwell T, Godhino J and Gott M (1995) *Tipping the Balance Towards Primary Health Care.* Avebury Press, Aldershot.

Roemer MI (1990) *Making Health Care Work for Society as We Move Towards the 21st Century*. Keynote Address: Nurses and Prescriptive Authority Conference, 5–7 October 1990, San Diego, California.

Salter B (1998) *The Politics of Change in the Health Service*. Macmillan Press, Basingstoke.

Shestowsky B (1997, ongoing) *The Dissemination and Utilization of Research Findings for Use by Nurses in Practice and Policy Development*. School of Nursing, McMaster University, Ontario.

Touche Ross (1994) Report of a study on nurse practitioners. In: L Harrison and H Neve (1996) *A Review of Innovations in Primary Healthcare*. The Policy Press, Bristol.

UKCC (1999) *A Higher Level of Practice*. Report of the consultation on the UKCC's proposals for a revised regulatory framework for post-registration clinical practice. United Kingdom Central Council for Nurses, Midwives and Health Visitors, London.

WHO (1978 and subsequent) *Alma Ata Declaration* (on Health For All). WHO Regional Office for Europe, Copenhagen.

WHO (1996a) *Nursing Practice*. Report of a WHO Expert Committee, Technical Report No 860. World Health Organisation, Geneva.

WHO (1996b) *Integration of Health Care Delivery*. WHO Technical Report Series 861. World Health Organisation, Geneva.

WHO (1997) *Health Care in Transition*. World Health Organisation, Geneva.

CHAPTER TWO

Talking about nursing

Marjorie Gott

> ... *if they are going to be able to use their unique skills set, they have to sell it; they have to make other people understand what it is that they are bringing* . . . (UK practitioner/educator)

Work carried out in the UK during the late 1980s indicated that nurses working in the community needed to make better strategic alliances for health, and to introduce new ways and patterns of working (Gott and O'Brien, 1990). However it was recognised that:

> *Current structures and patterns of working, together with extremely heavy workloads inhibit collaboration and innovation.*

In conceding that the UK community nursing workforce (health visitors, school nurses and district nurses) had underused skills and unrealised potential, Gott and O'Brien recognised the relatively minor power to effect change that these groups possessed, particularly as they were and remain fragmented rather than unified in professional development and purpose. Acknowledging that significant and sustained change was unlikely to come from these groups, Gott and O'Brien advocated new autonomous clinical roles and career structures for senior clinical nurses, urging that these roles be developed in partnership with other health professionals and be driven by clearly identified health and illness care demands generated by local communities. This belief is the fundamental premise upon which this book and its collection of case studies and analyses are based and was the starting point for a wider international debate with senior clinical nurses and educators working in other countries.

For over a decade, the principal author and editor of this book has been engaged in international nursing work (research, curriculum development) in universities and health departments in the United States and Australia. These connections and early informal discussions led to the growing belief that UK community nurses were not alone in the role insecurity that they felt and the underuse of nursing potential that they experienced. A focus for a study about nursing practice, policy and change emerged and a clear need for an exploration of these issues at this particular time was expressed.

Before embarking on this study and involving other nurses, senior nurses working in national (English National Board for Nursing, Midwifery and Health Visiting) and international (United Kingdom Central Council for Nursing, Midwifery and Health Visiting, Nursing Division, World Health Organisation/ Europe) organisations were contacted and the rationale and need for the book was discussed. It was established that the issues to be raised needed to be explored and that no one else was pursuing them at that time.

It was decided that the study should take place on three continents: Europe, North America and Australia. Identical briefing strategies were used for all countries. The next stage was to obtain nursing and nursing-related policy documents to explore statements about, and opportunities for, development of nursing practice. Initially these related primarily to the UK, but knowledge of these documents and their contents prompted the editor to brief authors in the US and Australia to take note of relevant policy documents in the countries about which they were to write.

Issues to be explored were arrived at after a series of semi-structured, focused interviews had been carried out by the principal author to further clarify areas for investigation and discussion. The interview schedule is shown in Box 2.1. The schedule was designed to gain views about:

- the current state of community/public health nursing
- the power that these nurses possess
- preparation for involvement in influencing service delivery and policy making
- shared learning (with other health professionals) and preparation for teamworking
- management of change in service delivery.

Following the interview, a response sheet was left with interviewees to reflect on and then return in a pre-stamped envelope to the investigator. Statements inviting responses were taken from either published research or policy documents. The response sheet is shown in Box 2.2.

Box 2.1: Interview sheet

Date: Location:
Contact details:

- explain and check out the purpose of the project
- explore/clarify issues of concern to them
- explore/clarify issues of concern to the interviewer
- collect grey data (course information/mission statements/job descriptions, etc.)
- ensure ongoing contact; offer them something in return.

What do you see as the main issues around Community/Public Health Nursing (PHN) right now/why do you feel this way?
(prompt if necessary):

in healthcare generally?

in PHNing in particular?

(prompt)
What about involvement of PHNs in policy making at locality level: does it exist, why/not?
(push them to cite an explanatory vignette)

Do you think that PHNs are prepared for involvement in health policy making?
(prompt)
academically

experientially

What kinds of skills would be useful?
(If not mentioned, prompt):
- managing change (record if they offer individual behaviour or community context/conditions)

- working with others to promote change; does any shared (non-nurse) learning/working occur/ratio?

- who do you think are the key actors in community/public health service decision making/why?

- (how) does this affect nurse involvement (helps/limits)?

- What changes do you see in the future (helps/limits)?

- Is there anything else you would like to add?

Thank you
Explain that a transcript of the data will be returned to them for verification/clarification

Box 2.2: Nurses and health policy

Read the following statements. Record your responses.
Write a few lines of explanation as to why you answered the way you did.

Change will depend on leaders in nursing practice...who are proactive in seeking opportunities for the development of nursing. Their efforts must be backed by political commitment for progress in nursing and by broad support from other professions.

comment

Nurses in positions of leadership must be able to influence the decision-making mechanisms that set priorities and allocate resources for healthcare.

comment

Public Health Nurses (PHNs) at present are not generally employed to be engaged with health policy making; they are employed to do what they are told by managers and administrators.

comment

The area of health change with which PHNs are most involved is that of seeking to change peoples lifestyles.

comment

PHNs as change agents are reactive rather than pro-active.

comment

Preliminary findings

Before presenting and discussing interview findings and responses it is necessary to make some comments about the interview process itself. The process is one with which the interviewer believed herself to be comfortable, having used this method frequently during the previous two decades in nursing. In this particular instance, however, she found it difficult and sometimes traumatic to carry out focused interviews. This is because by probing a particular issue it is possible to raise questions which subjects sometimes do not wish to address and this can quite deeply challenge their sense of coherence. In one interview in particular the investigator felt as if she had been in a war zone and needed space and distance to work through and account for the interviewee's position. And hers was not an isolated position; there were shades of it in other interviews; hers was simply more extreme because of the ideological dissonance she experienced as a nurse educator: being required to transmit to others ideologies, positions and skills she herself had either lost faith in or was powerless to enact. It became evident to the interviewer that many of the dilemmas individual nurses are facing or suppressing alone are fundamental and universal nursing dilemmas about which the profession itself is, at best, uncertain, and at worst, contradictory and divided.

The main findings from interviews and response sheet comments were fairly dispiriting. They showed a profession insecure and divided, which, although often articulate and politically aware, appeared rarely able to engage in shaping innovative nursing practice.

Nurses' relationship to shaping health policy was felt to be weak. This was particularly so for public health and other community nurses working in the US. Key actors in local decision making on health issues were said to be mayors, judges, elected officials and physicians. In the communication shown below the interviewer was requiring the interviewee, a nurse manager, to talk through how a community nurse might bring an unmet community need to their attention, and cites an instance based on a real local health issue:

Interviewer:

> *Say a nurse moves into a community and observes a health threat; say a Hispanic population with a high incidence of teenage pregnancies. What does she do, who does she work with?*

Interviewee:

> *That's a real difficult issue here. Normally you would go into the school but if you did that a lot of parents would get real upset. And then there's the Faiths (Churches) I guess they consider that the schools shouldn't be messing in issues that don't concern them. It's the family's business.*
>
> (Nurse manager, USA)

Whilst the above situation is an extremely difficult one for nurses to address, the tone of the exchange was reactive rather than proactive. The assumption was that nurses could do nothing. They certainly could not even begin to work on the issue with this type of leadership. Yet teenage pregnancy is a major social and health issue in the US and rates are disproportionately highest for teenage girls from disadvantaged groups. Promotion of health is an accepted nursing function; promotion of the health of teenage girls (the mothers and social shapers of future generations) should be a health promotion priority. Excellent projects, led by nurses, exist that do address this issue (McFarlane and Fehir, 1994; Laffrey, 1995; Brown *et al.*, 1999; Lambke and Kavanaugh, 1999). These should be known about and their benefits broadcast and sold politically. They then may stand a greater chance of local adoption and adaptation.

The tone of this Nursing Department's (1998) Strategic Plan was also passive and reactive, rather than proactive. Six domains of activity are delineated. They are:

1 To provide leadership in public health nursing (advancing nursing and the state/departments' interests within the profession, i.e. promoting and staffing a nursing leadership council).
2 To provide leadership in policy making by:
   • annually reviewing/updating the (State) Department of Health agency standards, manuals, policies and procedures
   • interpreting the Nursing Practice Act as it applies to public health nursing practice.
3 To participate in decision making as a member of nursing and multidisciplinary management teams:
   • serve on advisory committees, task forces and work groups
   • assess need, develop curricula, provide accreditation and evaluate the effectiveness of public health/community nursing.
4 To manage agency resources and information systems.
5 To develop coalitions with community organisations, health providers and business and consumer groups (all of the four interventions listed are couched in terms of co-ordination and collaboration).
6 To develop programmes that improve health.

Facing the future confidently was an issue for this manager and the nurses she leads.

Facing the future was also an issue for UK health visitors who probably receive more in the way of 'political awareness' education than most other community nurses. Talking about a student, an educator said:

> *Something which came to the fore this morning; one of them has listed in her weaknesses that need to be addressed the need to develop marketing skills for health visitors. This is something about which I feel fairly strongly, having just come from service. It's absolutely essential. General practitioners understand what district nurses do and they try to put health visitors under the same umbrella. I think health visitors are beginning to realise that if they're going to be able to use their unique skills set, they have to sell it; they have to make other people understand what it is that they are bringing and that it's different from what they've witnessed or inferred from health visiting practice. That seems to me a real hurdle . . . Increasingly I'm finding that's happening at practice level. People are having to have those debates with themselves and are having to take a stance.*

All nurses, not just health visitors, would benefit from better marketing skills. In developing these skills, nurses would need to follow through some challenging issues which they have previously sidelined, such as the mismatch between levels of preparation and practice, the value of clinical skills and their relationship with medicine and public health work.

Underuse and under-recognition of nursing skills are evident in the above quote and were also cited by other interviewees.

Opportunities for collaborative education and teamworking exist, but are fairly limited. Nurse educators in all three countries report initiatives where they provide shared learning opportunities which are generally well attended by nurses and social workers, but are extremely poorly attended by doctors.

Even highly visible nationwide schemes (USA Community–Campus Partnerships for Health, described in Chapter Six) report difficulties. A USA educator describes these, but also the benefits that come when shared learning does occur:

> *Most of the grantees that we worked with were interdisciplinary so they did have to work together, service learning was a good way of breaking down turf issues between medical*

*students and nursing students and pharmacy students. Hope-
fully if the faculty person sees these turf issues, they're going
to design a service-orientated course that allows all the
students to have equal participation. So we've seen examples
where the nursing students and the medical students are
working together but because of the medical students schedule they don't have to do as much and that has caused a rift,
so I talked to a nursing faculty at X University and she had
medical students from another university doing work with
her nursing students and she started the programme off and
she said: 'Each and every one of you . . . (she set the ground
rules and basically said) . . . medical students you will do just
exactly what the nursing students will do.' . . . Students that
have engaged in interdisciplinary service learning say that
service learning has helped them work more collaboratively;
that it helps diffuse some of those turf issues that had existed
earlier on.*

Poor attendance for shared learning is a situation the medical profession
and its educators need urgently to address. Primary healthcare, as we
now understand and seek to practise it, is not a one-man band. It
requires courtesy, respect and diffidence to work collaboratively for the
benefit of others. Doctors, it seems, still largely have not got the
message.

In addition to the medical profession's reluctance to engage in shared
learning, sometimes there is institutional opposition, from within the
nursing department itself. One very committed USA educator spoke of
her regret about this:

*Currently, no; there is no shared learning. It's a great concern
for me, and also a sadness. I think it should occur; in fact I
developed a course, a service-based interdisciplinary course,
but I wasn't able to get it funded (through the nursing
department) the meeting was awful, just awful. There were
these nine other people just staring at me as if I was mad . . .
it's just not on their wavelength. . . . This kind of multi-
sectoral working is a very low priority, no matter what they
say. They just give it lip service.*

The educator went on to talk about lack of teamwork, vision and
adaptability to community need:

*The problem is the Public Health Department doesn't know
what community health is. They see it still as individualistic; take the refugee clinic (from across the Mexican border),*

refugees are brought in at a time to suit the doctor ... even if they've just arrived at 4am in the morning. The doctor goes during normal working hours and takes all the records with him in the trunk of the car when he leaves ... and the nurse doesn't see anything wrong with that ... there's a lack of vision.

Reorientation of healthcare to serve individuals and communities was something that the senior nurse educators and practitioners were very aware of. Some were having success in changing practice:

We do things like getting the students to look at a major policy initiative and really explore it. You can take things like The Patients' Charter and look at the real implications of that ... and sometimes how bad a policy it is! We feel we are creating something for the students; we're getting them to think from the bottom up rather than the top down. And to look at policy and work it from where the patient is, and also to get people to do assignments in that area ... The Degree students are out there with a portfolio using real material ... I've got a student who's in a particularly rural area of X where patients, if you said 'You have to go to a Leg Ulcer Clinic (in town)' they would think that was like going to the moon. There's no way that they would have transport themselves, or even if you were to organise it they would go. Consequently the student thought that they were getting second-rate care and so she put the case to managers and that's been persued by the Health Trust to develop either a Leg Ulcer Clinic in that area, or look at training staff to give the care there.
(UK educator)

The need for more public health nurses and nurse practitioners (to give primary care, do risk reduction and health promotion work) was cited in all three countries. The following extract from the USA School of Nursing/Strategic Plan 1995–2000 is typical:

the projected demand for increased primary healthcare services focused on health promotion and disease prevention lead to a demand for new and expanding advanced practice nursing programmes. Further, hospitals will likely employ clinical nurse specialists to supplement the projected decline in the numbers of available resident physicians.

Education for practice

Education is the key to development of excellence in nursing practice, and thus improved healthcare services. Appropriate educational opportunities encourage the development of flexible and innovative best practice and a political awareness of how this can be advanced in a contextually sensitive collaborative way. According to WHO (1996):

> *Nursing education programmes [should be]:*
> - *based on the most recent assessment and forecasts of a country's health needs and of the nursing services required to meet them*
> - *problem based so as to promote the skills of critical thinking and problem solving*
> - *rooted in the philosophy of primary healthcare*
> - *founded on current research in nursing practice*
> - *culturally appropriate*
> - *multidisciplinary, where appropriate, to encourage shared learning and greater understanding between professions.*

In the early stages of planning this book, in addition to talking with senior nurses about nursing practice, policy and change, the lead author explored community nursing curricula (health visiting and district nursing) in the UK. These traditional forms of preparation far outweigh other forms of community/public health nurse preparation so it was believed to be important to get a sense of how radical and innovatory they were in preparing practitioners to operate in today's rapidly changing healthcare system. The English validating nursing body (English National Board for Nursing, Midwifery and Health Visiting) supplied a list of training institutions at which courses were offered and a one-in-three sample of curricula were obtained. Field visits were also made to three institutions.

Although this was a crude measure, it nevertheless provided an overview of which sets of issues and skills were valued and weighted highly and which received little or no formal (stated curricula) attention. It was found that curricula opportunities to develop skills for engaging in influencing health policy and managing change in practice were not given precedence, indeed sometimes went unmentioned. Lecturers working at one university, however, cited the validating body itself as a brake on progress: the submission they had originally presented to the board was seen as too radical and had to be watered down:

I think that in the course that is starting in September (1997) social policy is very much integrated. We don't actually have a module for social policy; it is integrated into the whole thing. We decided we didn't want a module; we've gone away from the trend in modules . . . it's interesting how much that was debated at the (ENB) Validation. It was felt it might get missed, but it's my subject area, I KNOW it's there in nearly every module. It's such a step forward because it's in everywhere. (offers the interviewer a copy of the submission document); *. . . Actually it was more radical than this, we have had to water it down for the approval process.*

(UK nursing lecturer)

With these findings in mind, authors invited to contribute to this book were asked to address education and validation issues when describing the case studies of advancing nursing practice that they were to present. They were also asked to think about political process and context because it was felt that these were areas that nurses were not generally engaged with and by:

Policy is a highly contested process and there's a lot of competing interests in it. Healthcare practitioners, if they are going to influence things in terms of PHC outcomes; working with people, need to understand that, and what I find is that the vast majority (of nurses) have no idea that policy is a political process or that they could actually influence it, or how they might do that. So we've run a (Masters in Contemporary Health Issues) course for two years now and in the beginning I think that people were like; 'what is this really dry kind of stuff?' You know; policy is hardly something that makes people excited . . . but I think that by showing them how those issues relate to their experiences in work practice, how it effects people in the community, how all those decisions are actually made, how the struggles actually manifest themselves, they start to see that there are ways that they can influence things and that if they're going to be effective healthcare practitioners, which we're aiming for them to be, if they don't understand the policy process and if they don't understand its political way and its contested nature then they're not going to be effective.

(Australian lecturer)

The need for case studies of good practice

Fragmentation of nursing services has been alluded to earlier, as has the difficulty nurses and other health service workers sometimes have in working together. Boelen (1998) comments:

> *Twenty years after the Alma Ata Declaration (1978), we still perceive the need for innovative health reform proposals powerful enough to attract and engage policy makers, health managers, the health professions, academia and consumers, in a collaborative pattern of work for the steady and sustainable improvement of quality, equity, relevance and cost effectiveness in health services. While convergence of efforts is an important prerequisite, stakeholders largely continue to express priorities and expectations that reflect their particular interests. Divergent agendas continue to exist and fragmentation in the health system has never been so pronounced.*

The way to bring health agendas and health practice together is to have nurses and other health professionals work on consumer-driven projects that can be explored and replicated as case studies of good practice. This is a sound and well-tested approach that has been advocated in Chapter One and was the method chosen for this project.

The decision to focus on good practice incidents was quite deliberate. It avoids focusing on the work of particular professional groups, and thus rivalries, but begins with a community's need for nursing services. By exploring what works, how and why, it is also possible to explore difficulties and obstacles surmounted. This is a much more valuable exercise than adding to a very large body of work citing difficulties and failures in the nurses' role.

Focusing on bottom up (needs driven) good practice also allows for exploration of across-the-board (treatment and care, health protection and health promotion) nursing activities that utilise and showcase the special skills of nurses and demonstrate their worth as frontline health workers in the community. What health policy makers and service purchasers and managers want and need to see are broadly applicable case studies of good practice in service delivery that work efficiently and effectively. Given the scale of population need and the dominant size of the nursing workforce, opportunity for development of innovative nursing practice is vast. The results of this strategy should yield useful information for practising nurses, managers, teachers and policy makers by addressing:

- what 'good practices' have been identified
- whether, and how they should be replicated
- what developments in teaching and preparation for practice need to occur.

The authors of the following chapters were selected to choose and describe case studies of good nursing practice that are of interest internationally and have potential for the development of nursing practice, nursing education and health policy in the future. During briefing, one author asked for more clarification about nurses and policy; did the editor mean policies affecting practice or practice affecting policies? The editor's reply is shown in full below as, in addition to helping the individual author, it illustrates a central tenet of this book; recognition of change, opportunity and contextual sensitivity:

> . . . you should address policies affecting practice AND practice affecting policies (I guess I see it as symbiotic). This can be bottom up (i.e. good practice gets disseminated more widely because there is a need and nurses can meet it), or top down (practice is extended or limited by change such as application of a new purchaser contract). I see it as a Big Picture/little snapshot thing. The Big Picture is the politico-economic context; the snapshots are the case study examples that work or don't work because of the local and the larger context.

There was regular two-way supportive contact between the principal and other contributing authors. At the case study drafting stage, authors were asked to comment on, in particular:

- a description of the service and the population to whom it is offered
- the policy context in which the nursing initiative is taking place (to include key actors and windows of opportunity)
- a review of the difference made to the population served
- roles and relationships with other service providers
- implications for nursing practice, nursing education and health policy making.

The case studies selected are presented in the next six chapters. The chapters are arranged in three sections; each section is preceded by a short introduction to the healthcare context in the country in which the case studies described are located. Perspectives taken are current, historic and the future. The first section (UK) showcases new practices and dilemmas; themes and issues raised here recur in the two following sections: nursing in the US, and nursing in Australia.

References

Alma Ata Declaration (1978) *Report of the International Conference on Primary Health Care*. World Health Organisation, Geneva.

Boelen C (1998) Unifying healthcare. *Changing Medical Education and Medical Practice* **June**: 22–3.

Brown HN, Saunders RB and Dick M (1999) Preventing secondary pregnancy in adolescents: a model program. *Health Care for Women International* **20** (1): 5–15.

Gott M and O'Brien M (1990) *The Role of the Nurse in Health Promotion: Policies, Perspectives and Practices*. Department of Health, London.

Laffrey SC (1995) *Empowering Individuals in CHCs to Take Responsibility for Their Health and Their Community From the Client Perspective*. Conference Speech, Community Health Centres, Centre of Health Care Reform. University of Montreal, Canada, 3–5 December.

Lambke MR and Kavanaugh K (1999) Nurses' description and evaluation of reproductive health counselling for adolescent females. *Health Care for Women International* **20**(2): 147–62.

McFarlane J and Fehir J (1994) De madres à madres: A community primary healthcare program based on empowerment. *Health Education Quarterly* **21**(3): 381–94.

WHO (1996) *Nursing Practice*. Report of a WHO Expert Committee, Technical Report No 860. World Health Organisation, Geneva.

The United Kingdom

Healthcare, health policy and nursing

Marjorie Gott

The National Health Service (NHS) was conceived as part of a radical public sector health and welfare package following the Second World War. It has undergone many reforms since then, but essentially remains a 'cradle to grave' service, free to all, centrally controlled and funded via general taxation. Its basic tenets are altruistic egalitarianism and involve guaranteed state provision of 'health' as the citizen's right. Any attempts to shift the duty of responsibility for health over the years have been highly politically charged and 'protection of our NHS' remains a central political issue at recurrent government elections (Salter, 1998).

Services are delivered by doctors, nurses, paramedics and related health and welfare professionals working in hospital and primary healthcare (PHC) settings. PHC is the first point of contact with the NHS for the vast majority of patients (99% of the population are registered with a general medical practitioner – GP). The PHC team comprises GPs, nurses and other professional staff who both provide direct service and act as gatekeepers for referrals to the hospital system. In common with other developed societies, up until the mid-1970s most NHS policy and practice was focused on secondary (hospital) care, but more recently there has been an intention to redistribute the ratio of resources (currently around 70% for hospital, 30% for PHC) in favour of primary care.

Significant changes in the NHS have occurred during the last two decades. Principle amongst these have been the growth of the private (for profit) sector as an alternative form of health provision, and the introduction of business management (Baggott, 1998).

Business sector management practices were imported into the NHS in the 1980s by the then Prime Minister, Margaret Thatcher, as part of a package of public sector reforms to make services more accountable, cost-effective and efficient (this in spite of the fact that, worldwide, the NHS was regarded as **the** model for effective and efficient health service delivery). Introduction of a whole new tier of (expensive) non-clinical managers into the NHS is now generally regarded to have been a failure, yet these and other 'market' measures remain, and have been adopted by the (now) socialist government. The Private Finance Initiative (PFI) for example has been retained as the way to finance the NHS building programme: irrespective of the fact that private companies investing in the PFI require at least a minimum return on their investment which means that, to meet this demand, future NHS services and hospital bed capacities will have to be cut. The PFI scheme is an attractive proposition for politicians who can be seen as busily and altruistically providing lots of 'improvements' and 'developments' to the NHS, however, in the longer term this is a deeply unattractive solution for the public, who will have to pick up the bills.

Short-term political expediency (money now for the NHS, not through rationing or charges) is putting at risk the integrity of the health service and its professional staff. Rationing does occur (covertly) and eventually some charges for some services are likely to be required (there is already a prescription charge for the able-bodied of working age). NHS staff are at the interface where principles meet resources. Honesty and solidarity with each other and with the public is the only viable way forward for nurses and doctors as they negotiate the increasing complexities and contradictions in a national health service which has no apparent limits but evident finite resources.

Retention of the market-driven purchaser/provider healthcare services division (introduced in the 1990 NHS and Community Care Act), although softened in scope from the divisive competitiveness of the Thatcher/Major regime, remains the mechanism for health service delivery. GPs have been given more power by measures that came into force in April 1999. They now lead primary care groups (PCGs) commissioning (purchasing) care for groups of patients of around 100 000. Budgets for hospital and community have been unified. There are financial incentives for areas that perform well and PCGs are able to use savings to improve services.

Another criteria that was introduced as part of the introduction of business management into the NHS was clinical audit of effectiveness. Unlike other changes, health service workers generally welcomed this move and doctors and nurses now, increasingly, audit their work. In addition, national standards are now being set and a National Institute for Clinical Excellence has been established (1999) to issue guidance on best practice to achieve clinical and cost-effectiveness.

Nurses and other health professionals

The medical profession, as in other western countries, has dominated healthcare and health policy during the 20th century. Subtle shifts in the status of nursing and the paramedic professions are evident at the turn of the century, however, due in part to changed public consciousness about the relative value of 'scientific' medicine and related high-technology care, and a revival of interest in public health, environmental safety, feminine value systems and alternative medicine.

In addition to the shift in status referred to above, nursing has several advantages. It is the largest single occupational group within the NHS, it has an unrivalled level of public support and (slowly) it is getting an increasing amount of autonomy. The group with most autonomy (midwives) has, during the 1990s, enjoyed increasing political support and many nurses see autonomous midwifery practice as a model for advanced clinical nursing practice in other specialist areas.

Nursing gained enhanced professional status in the 1980s due to both the creation of a new professional body and the relocation of nurse education from hospital-based schools of nursing into the higher education sector. Nursing is not an all-graduate profession in the UK, with many nurses not progressing beyond Diploma level. Regarding registration, in 1983 the United Kingdom Central Council for Nurses, Midwives and Health Visitors (UKCC) took over from the old General Nursing Council and brought nursing an enhanced degree of professional self-control. It is responsible for:

- determining nursing policy
- ensuring standards for registration
- specifying courses of nursing education
- investigating instances of alleged misconduct.

One of the most significant contributions the UKCC has made to the profession has been the post-registration education and practice (PREP) framework. Whilst this was visionary in its inception (requiring evidence of continued education of practitioners as they regularly [every three years] register their intention to practice), there is now a feeling that UKCC has 'lost the plot' with regard to recognising and credentialling advanced nursing practice. A recent report (JM Consulting 1999) proposes radical recommendations for change in regulatory frameworks and the establishment of a new Nursing and Midwifery Council to replace the UKCC and the four national boards. A new Strategy for Nursing document (DoH, 1999) also outlines the need for more open and flexible education and registration pathways for nurses. In the meantime, UKCC continues to deliberate on 'A higher level of practice' and 'specialist education' (UKCC, 1999a, b).

The reform of the apprenticeship system of nursing education that took place in the 1980s firmly located nurse preparation in the higher education sector and raised the status of the profession. Continuing education requirements are in place: these are to ensure that nursing practice is current and safe. There is a steady growth in the establishment of expert nurses (clinical nurse specialists, nurse practitioners, primary nurses), which is set to rise as politicians become increasingly aware of the economic and service benefits of employing nurses as the first point of contact in a re-orientated health service. Encouraging signs are the inclusion of nurses on primary care commissioning groups, the nationwide provision of a telephone healthline (NHS Direct), staffed by teams of specially trained nurses, and nurse-led 'walk-in' health centres.

Public health

Although there are health inequalities in terms of region, gender, class and ethnicity, the general standard of health today in the United Kingdom is high. The rate of infectious diseases in general has continued to fall, and, as in other western countries (due partly to greater longevity), rates of chronic disease have risen. Western diseases comprise cancers, coronary heart disease, hypertension and obesity and together account for 80% of disease mortality. Western diseases are associated with modern lifestyles and environments and are recognised as reversible, given better public health policies and practices.

There is now a broader based emphasis on public health in the UK. Following the 1997 general election in Britain and the end of 18 years of Conservative (capitalist) rule, changes in health policy were promised. Two months after taking up office the Health Secretary announced plans for 'health action zones' in inner cities. The action zones now exist, and bring together NHS bodies, local authorities, community and voluntary groups and local businesses to deliver change against targets, and to achieve measurable improvements in public health.

A parallel 'healthy public policy' initiative is the plan for a nationwide network of Healthy Living Centres. Again, the aim is to encourage broad-based alliances between health, local authority, NHS providers, leisure and welfare agencies and the business sector.

The public health approach has been strengthened but the power of vested interests (health businesses, hospital medical consultants) to resist change and consolidate their position remains a threat to democracy in healthcare. Nurses need to be aware of the agendas of key actors in health service decision making and to form alliances and develop practices to ensure the survival and furtherance of equitable and accessible care to meet the health and illness needs of the public they serve. The following two chapters illustrate how some nurses in the UK are doing this.

In Chapter Three, Naomi Chambers describes the differences nurse practitioners are making to the delivery of PHC services, and in Chapter Four, Margaret Bamford reports on the introduction of a nurse-led minor injuries unit, designed to serve the needs of a rural community.

References

Baggott R (1998) *Health and Health Care in Britain* (2e). Macmillan, Basingstoke.

DoH (1999) *Making a Difference*. Department of Health, London.

JM Consulting (1999) *Regulatory Frameworks Working Document*. Commissioned by UKCC (unpublished).

Salter B (1998) *The Politics of Change in the Health Service*. Macmillan, Basingstoke.

UKCC (1999a) *A Higher Level of Practice*. United Kingdom Central Council for Nursing, Midwifery and Health Visiting, London.

UKCC (1999b) *Standards for Specialist Education and Practice*. United Kingdom Central Council for Nursing, Midwifery and Health Visiting, London.

CHAPTER THREE

A UK nurse practitioner study

Naomi Chambers

> . . . what has happened here, particularly over the last couple or three years, is that we have recognised each other's abilities more, and each other's limitations, and the tasks that are carried out nowadays are much more related to the skills and the abilities of the person carrying them out.   (General Practitioner)

This chapter considers nurse practitioners in general in the UK, and examines a particular case study in Derbyshire where three nurse practitioners in general practice were appointed to their posts in 1990, two of whom are still there in 1999. The study gives a rare opportunity therefore to see the development of the role over a considerable time.

The research reveals that as well as yielding benefits to patient care, changes in nurse–doctor relations and greater job satisfaction for the nurses, undertaking this type of role extension can trigger a greater confidence on the part of nurses participating in local health service management and policy making.

The development of nurse practitioner models in the UK

There has been no nurse practitioner movement in the UK to compare with the movement in North America and elsewhere. Instead there has been a small number of interested individuals who have experimented with different models, and a growing acknowledgement from the professions, the academic institutions and government review bodies that nurse practitioners may have a significant part to play. As far as nurse practitioners in primary care are concerned, there is no one universally accepted definition. Britain's most famous nurse practitioner, and the architect of the first nurse practitioner course, run by the Royal College of Nurses (RCN), Barbara Stilwell, has identified six key functions of a nurse practitioner (Stilwell, 1991):

- provision of direct access service for patients
- comprehensive assessment including physical examinations
- discrimination between normal and abnormal findings
- organisation of appropriate screening programmes
- employment of relevant social and communications skills
- limited prescribing.

The evaluators of nurse practitioners working across 20 pilot sites at the beginning of 1992 provided a similar definition and added (Touche Ross, 1994):

- the responsibility for seeing medically unscreened patients
- the discretion to diagnose, refer and treat patients across a wide range of disorders.

A clearer picture of an emerging UK nurse practitioner role can be obtained by looking at the various models. A number of alternative nurse practitioner models exist.

The first is the doctor substitute. This model has had limited applicability in the UK with 99% of the population registered with a general medical practitioner. Not all groups have access to primary medical care, however. Barbara Burke-Masters was a doctor substitute in the 1980s for homeless alcoholics in London's East End who were not registered with a GP. A variant of this model are the triage nurses within accident and emergency departments; some also provide treatment, request X-rays and arrange discharge. The doctor substitute model has been mooted recently to overcome medical manpower difficulties. Within the hospital sector, there has been a concern about junior doctors' hours, and nurses have been proposed as a substitute to do some of the doctors' work, for example at night. Nurse triage projects within general practice, for example to deal with patients seeking same-day appointments, have been found to produce similar or better levels of output and quality at lower costs (Coopers and Lybrand, 1996).

The second is the model of doctor's assistant, taking referrals from the doctor and practising within protocols in an extended nursing role. This model already operates in UK, in the hospitals with the development of clinical nurse specialists and in primary care with practice nurses developing expertise in specific areas, including women's health, asthma and diabetes. The model fits well in primary care, since practice nurses are, by and large, employed by the doctors with whom they work. But there is also evidence that some practice nurses would like to, and others already are, working more autonomously than this model would suggest, for example by determining and prioritising their own programme of work.

The third model is that of the nurse as an alternative first point of contact. This model offers to the public the choice of nurses or doctors as a first port of call when they have a health problem. These nurses have the authority to examine, diagnose and treat, following protocols agreed with the doctors, where appropriate, as well as utilising a holistic model of care, with a health advice and promotion focus. Midwives operate in this way: they practise autonomously, they are increasingly used as a first point of contact by women with a query in pregnancy, they can refer directly to obstetricians and they manage straightforward deliveries. Health visitors, in principle, also work autonomously. Within the practice setting, Stilwell and Restall worked liked this in the 1980s and Kaufman and many others in the 1990s, and the RCN-franchised nurse practitioner training course promotes this model (Stilwell, 1988; Kaufman, 1996).

Most recently, the Labour government has initiated NHS Direct, a 24-hour telephone helpline staffed by nurses, launched in three areas in March 1998 and planned to cover the whole country by the year 2000. Early indications suggest that callers are using the service not so much for general health information, but for advice on what to do about symptoms they or their families are experiencing. The nurses, chosen for their experience of independent decision making and the quality of their communication skills, use sophisticated clinical decision support system software and question callers closely about their symptoms. Of the first 790 calls to the service in Newcastle, in the industrial North of England, 95% were symptom-based enquiries, that is help for an immediate health problem, 37% resulted in self-care, 6% needed urgent care and 2% required an emergency (999) response. Nurses responded to the remainder of calls with a range of help, including recommending a visit to the surgery, contacting out-of-hours GP services, and information and advice. In short, the public are using this new pilot service as an alternative first point of contact (Greenwood, 1998).

The predominant features of this model of the nurse practitioner as an alternative first point of contact for primary healthcare are likely to be the most appropriate for the UK primary healthcare environment, where teamwork in primary healthcare is being encouraged and where nurses are increasingly rejecting the handmaiden role. It conforms with the current public expectation for direct access to their family doctor, whilst allowing patients to see another health practitioner if they do not want treatment utilising a predominantly medical approach. The model of alternative first point of contact nurse practitioners can be enhanced, however, by borrowing from the other models described above. A measure of substitution is likely to be both feasible and desirable, for example, nurse practitioner appointments may be offered when doctors' appointments are fully booked, or a doctor has had to cancel a surgery. The doctor's assistant model has worked successfully in the relationship between practice nurses and family doctors, and elements from it may be useful as the nurse practitioner role in primary care emerges.

Training and preparation of nurse practitioners

Nurse practitioner courses are now being introduced all over the UK. By 1997 there were some 300 qualified nurse practitioners and similar numbers in educational programmes leading to a nurse practitioner qualification (Johnson, 1997). Levels of study vary from Diploma to Masters Degree, and course content varies between institutions. In addition, many courses advocate a GP mentor for trainee nurse practitioners as well as clinical supervision from within nursing. Some nurses have chosen to develop the role through bespoke training and development, without seeking the formal qualification. The main cause for concern is that the regulatory body for nurses, the UKCC, has yet to recognise the title or role. This means that the term 'nurse practitioner' is not a recognised nursing role at either specialist or advanced practitioner level. As Campbell (1997) argues, in doing this the UKCC invite the criticism that they have failed to meet their duty to protect the public by ensuring that all nurse practitioners are appropriately educated and experienced to take on such a role.

Triggers and barriers to the development of the UK nurse practitioner

Ironically, in view of the UKCC's stance on nurse practitioners, the main professional liberator for nurses in the last decade has been the adoption of *The Scope of Professional Practice* by the UKCC in 1992. This removed the major inhibitor which had been that any extension of role required official 'certification', preventing nurses from fulfilling their potential for the benefit of patients. Now the requirement is that nurses' scope of professional practice can be adjusted or enlarged as long as certain principles concerning patients' safety, personal competence, appropriateness of delegation and collaborative working are adhered to (UKCC, 1992).

Whilst *The Scope of Professional Practice* has legitimised nurse practitioner work, increasing pressures faced by GPs have at last improved, for pragmatic reasons, the acceptability, to their medical colleagues, of nurses running their own surgeries. Some 20 years ago, in research carried out in the late 1970s, Bowling found that only one quarter of doctors were in favour of the nurse carrying out the initial consultation in the surgery (Bowling, 1981). By 1993, 94% of family doctors in one study were in favour of patients being able to refer themselves directly to a nurse (Robinson *et al.*, 1993). Low morale amongst GPs facing unprecedented demands from the public in an open-access service is widespread, and there are increasing concerns about recruitment into general practice.

On top of patient demand, successive NHS reforms have brought general practitioners into the centre stage of health policy implementation, from the advent of fundholding through to GP commissioning, and most recently with the advent of PCGs , which all practices must to some degree participate in and cooperate with. PCGs, which generally encompass a population of 75 000–150 000, are charged with improving the health of the local population, commissioning hospital care and community nursing services and driving up the quality of primary care. Each PCG has seven GPs on the board, and the overwhelming majority have a GP chair. Whilst guardedly welcoming the prospect of being in the driving seat, GPs have expressed reservations about the amount of time out of general practice which this latest reform entails. Notwithstanding this concern, the government has already expressed a desire for some PCGs to progress to Trust status, which, as separate bodies from the health authority, will have full budgetary responsibilities and provide a comprehensive range of primary and community services.

The government has also quietly supported the development of the nurse practitioner role, from an initial definition and recommendation in the Cumberlege Report of 1986 through to the funding of pilot projects and evaluations, such as the one in South Thames (Touche Ross, 1994) and nurse-led practice projects as part of the Primary Care Act pilot scheme launched in 1998. Project funding and quiet approbation rather than a big policy push has been the government's stance, although a shift can be detected since the general election of 1997, with the advent of NHS Direct, the new telephone service staffed by nurses mentioned above, and the Health Secretary's proviso (Crail, 1998) that an increase in medical student numbers will be accompanied by discussions with the medical profession and others:

> . . . about the future shape of the healthcare workforce . . . [including] such issues as productivity and skill substitution.

It could be argued that the government's position, which could be summarised as approval without commitment, whilst encouraging brave individuals and practices, is also a main barrier to a wholesale development of the nurse practitioner role across the country. Similarly, the UKCC's stance is not helpful. The failure of the UKCC to recognise the nurse practitioner title is no mere oversight, nor can it be ascribed to the fact that the term 'nurse practitioner' itself is woolly, ambiguous and misleading; it probably is – although no one has thought of a better one. The UKCC's approach is no less than a reflection of many nurses' and doctors' own sense of ambiguity about a job which increasingly looks like a potent medley of their very separate professions.

A project which focused on the patients and professionals in three practices in Derbyshire in the North Midlands of England examined this issue of how the new nurse practitioner role affected inter- and intra-professional relations. The project also evaluated the impact of the new role on patients' experience of care at the surgery.

Derbyshire nurse practitioner project

The nurse practitioner model used in the Derbyshire project drew mainly from the one, described above, which has the nurse as alternative first point of contact for patients in primary care. This professional is:

- an experienced nurse with appropriate additional qualifications who offers primary healthcare consultations on undifferentiated health problems as an alternative first point of contact to going to see the family doctor
- a nurse to whom patients can go for diagnosis, treatment and advice for minor illness and for other health matters which patients may consider are appropriate for a nurse consultation

- a member of the primary healthcare team who works closely with other colleagues, especially the family doctor, and whose work is guided but not bound by protocols
- a nurse who largely focuses on a holistic nursing approach to healthcare but who draws from the medical model of health and illness where appropriate.

Three volunteer practices in Derbyshire were chosen from 19 who initially expressed interest. A common job description was drawn up for the three part-time nurse practitioners (ten hours per week), each funded at 100% for two years at (higher salary) Grade H. The project ran from 1990 to 1993, with the nurses in post from late 1990. Two were existing practice nurses who chose to extend their role and their hours, the third was a new recruit. The nurse practitioners had booked appointments, worked from a consulting room, and were able, within protocols, to decide on treatments including prescriptions, although a doctor's signature was always obtained, as required by law in the UK. The three practices had broadly similar characteristics, although geographically apart, serving a mixture of suburban and semi-rural populations with a predominance of white Caucasian working class, some hill-farming communities and some relatively prosperous middle-class commuting households. A follow-up visit to all three practices was paid in 1998 to find out what had happened since the completion of the project. The broad aim of the project was to utilise nursing skills more fully, enable GPs to practise their medical skills more extensively, and provide greater choice for patients. The research questions were the impact of the new role on patient satisfaction and on the primary healthcare team, hoping to come to a view about the potential for the future expansion of nurse practitioners in the UK. The project and associated research is described in more detail elsewhere (Chambers, 1996, 1998).

The main findings from patient surveys and focus groups with the health professionals in 1991–92 covered a number of themes, relating to the consultation experience, the organisation of primary care services and professional implications for doctors and nurses.

The patient consultation

Although the three nurse practitioners had the same job description, the content of their work varied as their role developed, however there was a common core which was the alternative first-point-of-contact surgery consultation service. In all three cases however, their work ran the gamut from minor illness treatment to health promotion.

In one of the practices, the nurse practitioner's clinical workload focused largely on the management of acute minor illness in adults and children, including chest and ear complaints. In a practice with a shortage of available doctor appointments, the nurse had busy surgeries with short consultation times. This nurse also began to specialise, and worked in more depth in the area of women's health and the menopause.

In the second practice, where the nurse was based at the branch surgery, which was relatively quiet in comparison with the main surgery belonging to the practice, the nurse ran health promotion and chronic disease management clinics as well as the undifferentiated open-access nurse practitioner surgeries, which ran concurrently with the visiting doctor's surgery consultations. The nurse began to build a close relationship with some of the regular patients because of the small size of the branch surgery, its catchment population and because the visiting doctors changed, whilst she was the familiar face. This nurse also developed a specialist interest in the management of asthma, which later led to a research and training role in this area.

In the third practice, the nurse also delivered health promotion and chronic disease management services, as well as the nurse practitioner consultation surgeries. The practice placed a strong emphasis on not drawing a clear line between these. As a consequence, this nurse's consultations often combined, in one episode, the management of a minor infection with counselling about a more long-term health problem. The nurse's clinical workload varied according to the availability of the doctors as there was not generally a shortage of doctor appointments in this practice, except during illness and leave.

What did the patients think about the nurse practitioners in the Derbyshire project? Postal questionnaires were sent twice to the three volunteer practices and to three matched control practices – once before the nurse practitioners started surgeries and then 18 months later. A total of 2400 questionnaires were mailed, and, with one reminder, a response rate of 76% was attained. The first finding worthy of note was that the nurse practitioners had achieved a reasonable depth of penetration into the population of the research practices, with nearly one in five of the respondents reporting having consulted her at least once, and a quarter of that group having consulted her more than once. This suggests a degree of acceptability which does not appear to come from the nurse acting as a doctor substitute, since access to doctor appointments was already very good. The nurse practitioner option was more popular for women than it was for men. Those respondents who did consult the nurse practitioner gave statistically significant higher satisfaction scores for the nurse in comparison with the doctor, using the four parameters of listening, explaining, information and time. Other research on patient satisfaction ratings for nurse practitioners corroborate this finding (Office of Technology Assessment, 1986; Touche Ross, 1994; Poulton, 1995). One hypothesis was that the advent of the nurse practitioner would free up time for doctors and allow them to concentrate on the patients who presented with clinically more complex conditions, thus resulting in a higher patient satisfaction for doctor consultations. In fact, although the dissatisfaction score with doctors in the research practices did drop, the results were not statistically significant.

Because of the research method chosen, the study could not examine why patients would choose to see a nurse practitioner, although further information is available from a qualitative study undertaken later in one of the practices (Chambers, 1995) involving the use of focus groups. Four main sets of views emerged. First, some participants had had experience of the nurse practitioner, and expressed confidence in the service: she knew what she was talking about, and called the doctor in if she was not sure about something. A second strand of opinion was that it was a worthwhile role, particularly to relieve pressure on the doctor. This suggests that the nurse as doctor substitute is at least partially acceptable. A third view was that the role was unknown and they were interested in finding out more, particularly how she could be consulted as a first point of contact. Fourth, there were some more wary participants who wanted information and reassurance that the nurse was appropriately trained, for example, this lady (Chambers, 1995):

> . . . Why do they put you in to see her when she is not a qualified doctor? I don't know what her qualifications are . . . my experience with [the nurse] is in the family planning clinic and with my blood pressure . . . and then I came for my ear or something and I thought: what is she looking in my ear for? . . . you've got an image of what a nurse does and you think that she is not qualified to diagnose anything else . . . we are not given enough information . . . when you think of a doctor, you know they have been through all those years of training . . . but if they gave us more information on what a nurse could do . . .

The study suggests that having trust in the nurse's professional standards of care is an important factor in the patient's decision to choose to see her, and not having that trust, because of a certain view about what nurses 'do', and in the absence of other information, can be a barrier.

The focus groups with the health professions offered an insight into how the nurse practitioner consultations differed from GP consultations. The doctors and nurses agreed that the nurse provided the opportunity for a more relaxed consultation, with a lesser likelihood of a prescription as an outcome, and the choice of another woman practitioner (in each of these three practices, there was at the time only one part-time woman doctor). The comments volunteered by respondents at the end of the postal questionnaire included valuing continuity and the opportunity to consult with someone of the same gender. Two of the nurse practitioners mentioned a growing confidence on the part of patients as they got to know her. Patients positively chose to see someone who had an understanding, perhaps through a greater overlap of common experiences, of their lives, but whom they could also trust as a competent professional person.

The organisation of primary healthcare services

One of the aims of the Derbyshire project was to see whether an additional nurse practitioner service would ease the pressure of demand for surgery appointments, reduce waiting times in the surgery and free up time for doctors to concentrate on patients with medically complex problems, while the nurse was seeing some of the patients presenting with minor illness. In fact, accessibility for non-urgent doctor appointments, and waits in the surgery, as measured by the patient questionnaire, did not improve significantly after the nurse practitioner started work. No other study has addressed this question precisely, but Touche Ross (1994) found that there was a tendency for the overall rate of consultations to rise with the introduction of nurse practitioners and there is also evidence in the US literature that consultations rise in these circumstances (Holmes *et al.*, 1976). The presence of the nurse practitioner may enable additional patients to be seen, thus meeting a 'care gap', but demand to see the doctor may not decrease and, indeed, the presence of the nurse practitioner may stimulate demand to see the doctor.

Another of the underlying propositions around which the project was conceived was that the introduction of another health professional offering additional surgery appointments would allow doctors to concentrate on the clinically more complex cases, which were more appropriate for their training, and would more closely suit their style of consulting. This would improve patient satisfaction with the medical consultation. The patients' survey results did not bear this out: the overall level of patient satisfaction did not improve in the research practices. Does this mean that the potential for doctors to improve on their patient satisfaction rating is limited? The results suggest that, by itself, adding the nurse practitioner to the pool of surgery consultation labour will result in neither improved access to appointments (they will still all be filled) or improved patient satisfaction with consultations provided by the doctors. One further point on this issue concerns the time that the nurse practitioner was available. The nurse practitioners were only able to offer ten additional hours of consulting time in each of the research practices (which comprised three, four and five doctor partners). It is possible that if the nurses had been full-time, offering 30 or so additional consulting hours, the redistribution of work, with the doctors assuming a greater proportion of the clinically challenging cases, would begin to take place, with the potential for improved patient satisfaction.

The doctors in the focus groups from the three research practices did not themselves feel that they had more time after the nurse practitioners were introduced. In terms of workload distribution, some felt that they were not doing anything very different from before, but that the nurse practitioner was enabling more patients to be seen. This supports the proposition that a nurse practitioner in primary care may be exposing and meeting the 'care gap' described earlier. Only in one of the practices, where the nurse practitioner operated a service at the branch surgery, did the doctors feel that they were far less busy and seeing a change in their work profile – seeing fewer children and patients with minor acute illness and gynaecological problems.

Doctors discussed many times the lack of control they had over their time, and highlighted the paradox of ready availability to patients with the need to adhere to the fixed time for meetings. These were the owners and directors of their enterprise, but they were finding that role difficult to reconcile with being first-point-of-contact practitioners. Allocating additional nurse practitioner appointments did not turn out to be an opportunity for them to take on something new or to deliver higher quality care. Given that patients signalled in the research that the style of the nurse practitioner consultation was more acceptable than their doctor's, is it time for doctors to let go a little of this 'first-point-of-contact' care, as they have in health promotion and some chronic disease management (to practice nurses) and in maternity care (to midwives) in order to step back, see where primary care is going, and regain some control over their enterprises and their lives?

A potential gain for patients in doctors' letting go might be the development of the patient–nurse relationship as an alternative to the doctor–patient relationship, the closeness of which has been described as a mirage (Balint *et al.*, 1993). In a discussion about doctor–patient relationships, Miles (1991) describes the clash between two kinds of expertise: on the one hand there is the professional expertise, based on general rules and categories, learned during training; and on the other hand there is lay expertise, built from personal experience and that of the social group. Nurses, if allowed, may be able to bridge the gap between these sets of expertise by offering to patients an understanding and insight developed from their advocacy role, as well as offering professional care from their clinical skills repertoire.

Professional implications for doctors and nurses

How far doctors are willing to let go and nurses are keen to push themselves forward was explored in the third area covered by the research, which was the impact of the nurse practitioner role on the doctors and nurses involved. The major concern emanating from the focus groups was the question of training. At the time there were no 'tailor-made' nurse practitioner courses available either locally or nationally, so there was a considerable time investment for the practices. As well as sitting in on surgery consultations, the development of protocols necessitated one-to-one tutorials with the doctor mentor; these had been fruitful, but one of the practices was doubtful whether they had the organisational capacity to train a nurse practitioner all over again. There was a further concern that external training courses for nurse practitioners, whilst conferring a recognised and portable qualification, would not be sufficient to engender trust in the doctors employing a nurse practitioner. What are doctors looking for in their new nursing colleagues? They want to be convinced that these are professionals who will not let them or themselves down. A local solution to the training problem might be a combination of the externally provided and validated course, such as the one now franchised by the RCN, with practice-based training with a GP mentor, in order for the doctors in the practice to develop confidence in sharing clinical decision making with a non-medical colleague.

The issue of inter-professional trust was debated at length in the focus groups. The nurse practitioners reported that over time, the doctors with whom they worked became more trusting and relationships became more relaxed. The doctors described the effect of having a nurse sitting in on consultations as making them think more deeply about what they were doing, and having to justify decisions. Changes in relationships affected the other nurses in the primary healthcare team too, the district nurses, health visitors and practice nurses. As one doctor put it:

> *. . . this is a continuum for the days of the 1965 Charter . . . before that time, doctors did everything, and the nurses were designed to help and to do things for the doctor . . . what has happened here, particularly over the last couple or three years, is that we have recognised each other's abilities more, and each other's limitations, and the tasks that are carried out nowadays are much more related to the skills and the abilities of the person carrying it out.*

How did the arrival of the nurse practitioner affect the other nursing members of the team in the Derbyshire project? It was agreed that there was role overlap, particularly between the practice nurse and nurse practitioner, and in one practice they had come to the conclusion that the nurse practitioner/practice nurse distinction was artificial. The nurses pointed out similarities with the way in which patients used practice nurses, district nurses and health visitors to get more information and advice about health problems. There had been some friction in one of the practices with the health visitor feeling that the nurse practitioner was doing in the surgery what she was doing in the home, but the dynamics within the nursing team changed, and by the second focus group, the health visitor in that practice reported that they were working together, and doing whatever each most preferred, with the skills they had got and the time available. In fact, in two of the practices, because they were hard-pressed and short-staffed, the health visitors had begun to take advantage of the availability of the nurse practitioner. They had found that their clients welcomed the opportunity to see a nurse at the surgery without having to worry about whether their child's problem was 'serious' enough for the doctor. The nurse practitioner had also acquired useful skills, for example, in sounding chests to see whether an infection had cleared.

The practice nurses in two of the practices were mildly envious of the attention and status accorded to the nurse practitioner. One made it clear that she would have become the practice 'expert' in menopause problems if the nurse practitioner had not come along. Another felt that she was already operating in an extended role as an alternative first point of contact. She was also concerned that the particular nurse practitioner model was tending too much towards the 'medical model', apeing what doctors did and not practising nursing.

Two of the nurse practitioners themselves expressed concerns about being a sort of 'second-class doctor' or 'plumber's mate'. They were, however, unequivocally enthusiastic about their work and their new responsibilities. They were clear about the differences between their scope of practice as practice nurses and as nurse practitioners providing a general surgery service. The move towards greater autonomy in professional practice had not been painless. They described their new work as much more taxing. All three had worried in the early days about missing an important symptom or making other mistakes. Although a significant proportion (in one practice it was about 50%) of nurse practitioner consultations resulted in drug treatment, and the nurses were not able legally to sign prescriptions, they seemed to cope with the minimum fuss and inconvenience to patients by arranging for one of the doctors, during surgery, to sign a prescription on their behalf between seeing patients.

The study demonstrated that the nurses as a whole were conscious of hierarchy and status, sensitive about a 'supernurse' model and wary of a 'second-class doctor' model. But, because patients were clearly benefiting, there was an acceptance, along with their medical colleagues, of the nurse practitioner acting as a first-point-of-contact health professional and also an acceptance of the new tasks of history taking, examination, diagnosis and management that the new role necessarily brought with it.

A 1998 update on the Derbyshire project

Taped interviews with doctors and nurses from the three research practices took place in September and October 1998 and with the nurse practitioner who had moved away in December 1998. Two of the practices still retained the same nurse practitioner from 1990. The third practice had a new nurse practitioner, who had been a practice nurse at the time of the project. The original nurse practitioner for this practice was back in Derbyshire at a different practice with a nurse management role.

The main questions asked during the interviews were as follows.

- Has the model of nurse as alternative first point of contact changed since 1992?
- Does the model help nurses to realise their potential, and if so how?
- Does the model provide patients with a different and/or better service, and if so how?
- What impact does the nurse practitioner role have on the doctors' work and on doctor/nurse relations?

Changes since 1993

In one practice, the model used, as well as the postholder, had not significantly changed since 1993. This practice had from the beginning used the nurse practitioner surgeries more consciously to alleviate the doctors' workload, rather than as a complementary service for patients, in other words borrowing more heavily from the doctor substitute model, without denying patients access to a doctor. The profile of patients coming to the nurse's surgeries had shifted slightly away from, although was still predominantly, acute minor illness. The nurse had also extended her clinical responsibilities with regard to referrals, which she now did herself to the hospital specialists for radiography, gynaecology, ear nose and throat, and the breast clinic. The nurse practitioner hours had increased from 15 to 29, and she had her own consulting room. She had completed a Nurse Practitioner Diploma course at Manchester University, followed by an honours degree, and she had taken on new management responsibilities, which are discussed further below.

The second practice still had the nurse practitioner (the same postholder) as alternative first point of contact, but had added a new role: the nurse practitioner was the first point of contact for on-call matters; that is, home visit requests and urgent advice from midday to midnight. This was the practice where they had decided that the nurse practitioner/practice nurse distinction was artificial, and the full-time nurse ran nurse practitioner surgeries during part of the week as well as carrying out more traditional practice nurse functions, such as health promotion and chronic disease management. As part of the surgery extension being built at the time of the visit this nurse practitioner was having her own consulting room constructed.

The third practice, where the original nurse practitioner left in 1993, had a new nurse practitioner who, as well as performing the traditional practice nurse role, for part of her working week, has been, since April 1998, the first point of contact for patients requesting a same-day appointment after 11.30 am. The idea was a triage system for managing calls, and the nurse estimated that about 90% of the requests were managed, either over the telephone or by a consultation at the surgery, by her without need for onward referral to a doctor. This nurse expressed similar concerns which had surfaced six years earlier with the others about her fear, in the newness of the extended role, of missing something or making a mistake.

The nurses from all three practices expressed continuing enthusiasm for their work. Two of the practices had new partners who had joined since the role had been developed, who were both impressed by the nurse practitioners' expertise and ability to participate in clinical decision making, described thus by one of them:

> I was very pleased to see that . . . you were not following orders or very strict guidelines . . . I was very impressed that you weren't just running down very strict alleyways . . . I was impressed by the breadth of cases you were covering . . . the stuff you were prescribing was correct . . . the standard of practice is far better than about 20–30% of GPs in Britain at the moment, simply because you have applied thought to the process of seeing the patient.

The stories from these three practices suggest that the nurse practitioner's extended skills in clinical assessment, diagnosis and management were now being used more for doctor substitute purposes than they had been at the inception of the Derbyshire project, whilst still retaining the essence of an alternative first point of contact, since direct access to doctors was not being denied. The fact that two of the original postholders were still there, with the third practice adopting a variant of the nurse practitioner role with a new postholder, indicates an enduringly viable and acceptable model.

Nurse practitioners and primary care management

The two original nurses now also had a management role within the practice, one managing the two practice nurses and participating fully in practice management meetings with the partners and the practice manager; the other co-ordinating all nursing activity, across practice nursing, district nursing and health visiting, steering a well-developed, integrated nursing team. In the former practice, the nurse practitioner was the nurse representative on the local subcommittee for the PGC to which the practice belonged, and she also led the local nurse group, and therefore had taken on responsibilities for developing and maintaining good relations with the community nurses in the locality. In the third practice, the new nurse practitioner was taking an active interest in the development of PCGs. She explained how her Nurse Practitioner Masters Course had opened her eyes and stimulated her awareness of nursing and health policy politics. She reported that she went to a number of local primary care meetings in her own time because of a 'huge interest' in what was going on. As well as a desire to sort out integrated nursing locally, her interest also extended to national issues:

> *I'd like to work with the UKCC to shape the future because I feel that the UKCC is holding back . . . they won't take a decision about the title of nurse practitioner, they won't take a decision about nurse prescribing . . . so many things that they have been sitting on the fence about.*

One of the practice nurses in the research practices who had not opted for the extended role as a nurse practitioner was also studying for a Masters Degree in Primary Health Care. Her sights were now set on getting involved in the local PCG, perhaps on the board.

These nurses were demonstrating an eagerness and assertiveness to participate in decision making about primary care issues far beyond the concerns of the practice nurse treatment room, whilst still retaining and developing their clinical expertise. What were the triggers? It appears that they were twofold: the 'permission' given by their extended role, but also the experience of higher level education courses with exposure to the power politics in nursing and medicine.

Nurse practitioners and patient care

The 1998 update did not include any patient surveys, but information was obtained from the practices about what they considered to be the continuing benefits for patients of the role. As before, there was evidence from all three sites that patients particularly liked the speedy access to a health professional, which the availability of nurse practitioner appointments provided. Over the years, the patients from the two practices where the same nurse practitioner postholder had remained had become more aware of the role and were using the nurse practitioner consultation for more than minor acute illness, particu-larly for women's health and counselling. Another asset was the time to listen to patients properly, which doctors felt that they did not have. There was also the opportunity to share a problem with someone who was not a doctor. One of the practices with the longstanding nurse practitioner indicated that, in addition to the minor acute illness, some of the nurse practitioner's workload involved patients who would only go to her, in other words, her own 'caseload' of patients who had developed a loyalty to the nurse rather than to one of the doctors.

The conclusions from this update as far as patient benefits are concerned remain the same as in the original study: choice, access, a more relaxed consultation style, and the opportunity for women to consult with a woman were all important.

Nurse practitioner role and doctor–nurse relations

In one of the practices there was a feeling that the nurse practitioner saw very much the same mix of patients as the doctors, with perhaps slightly more patients with gynaecological problems than the male partners. In the other two practices, the doctors felt that they were seeing much less acute minor illness when the nurse practitioner was consulting. Doctors at the practice where the nurse practitioner was first on call from midday to midnight on some days felt the difference, particularly the fact that they were not being disturbed. Doctors from the practice who had developed the same-day triage system described how their afternoon surgeries were much lighter and that they were able to spend more time with their patients to get to the bottom of things. There was also a sense that they were managing more clinically complex cases than before:

> *you can see people properly as well . . . if they come with something complicated . . . you buy time in all sorts of ways in this job . . . with a blood test or a prescription . . . or a 'come back and see me next week' . . . whereas when you know you haven't got lots of people waiting outside you can sit down and sort them out so they don't come back next week . . . so there is a long-term benefit . . . one of the things I have found over the past few years is that I have had to lengthen my appointment times because I couldn't keep up any more . . . all the easy stuff . . . the blood pressures . . . we don't get those any more . . . we see complicated things . . . people on very complex drugs . . . they would have been seen on a regular basis [at the hospital] every two months . . . [now] they may be seen every six months . . . and if there is a problem they come and see us.*

This comment suggests that one of the hypotheses from the original project; that if doctors let go of some of the first-point-of-contact work, they might spend more time with clinically more challenging issues may now, in contrast to the earlier findings, be coming true.

The interviews with the practices suggested again that the new role facilitated a strengthening of mutual respect between the nurses and the doctors. The latter, particularly the ones who had recently joined the practice, were impressed, as was discussed earlier, by the clinical expertise of the nurse practitioner. The new nurse practitioner, in the practice which had developed the triage system for requests for same-day appointments, described how her respect grew enormously when she realised the scale of the differing problems that patients presented to GPs, all of which the doctor was supposed to know how to tackle, or whom to go to.

Following on from this discussion about inter-professional relations, the interviews also covered the issue of nurses in partnership with doctors. Two of the practices were clear that they would go for a more even balance of nurse practitioners to doctors. One reason given was that they were more amenable to protocols and guidelines and that it was therefore easier to run the organisation with the key participants all working in the same way. Another reason given was that nurse practitioners were as effective as and cheaper than doctors. The main barrier was perceived to be the basic practice allowance and capitation fees, part of the method of paying family doctors in the UK, which are only payable to doctors, not to nurses. All three nurses cited the lack of prescribing rights as a major hindrance to their personal development and credibility as full partners. The changes in the UK law from April 1999, which allow some nurses limited prescribing rights, do not go nearly far enough either in terms of the formulary, or the kinds of nurses who are allowed to prescribe.

The study demonstrated that not all nurses would want an extended role in the form of nurse practitionership. It has already been noted that one of the practice nurses in one of the research practices was aiming, as the next stage in her personal and professional development, for participation in the wider PCG rather than developing an extended clinical role. In the practice which had developed a triage system for requests for same-day appointments, the practice nurse was clear that she did not want to be bullied into participating in the triage until she was personally and professionally ready, which she felt that she was definitely not at the time of the update interviews.

One of the original nurse practitioners from the Derbyshire project who had left in 1993, and who was also interviewed as part of the update, had moved on from wanting to focus solely on alternative first-point-of-contact work, which she felt many practice nurses already did, sometimes in the form of triage. This nurse had left her practice in 1993, and had for a short time worked at another local practice as a practice nurse, but also developing the nurse practitioner role and running two nurse practitioner-style surgeries a week. For family reasons she then moved away and took a post as an asthma specialist in a hospital. The family moving once more, her current post was as a nurse manager in a large, busy, city practice, as well as being a regional asthma trainer. Her concern was now to develop practice nursing, not as a doctor substitute, nor as an alternative for acute minor illness, but in the areas of women's health, ear nose and throat, and chronic disease management, and to challenge, through the nurses, the primary/ secondary care boundaries. This nurse was, like the two described earlier, also studying for a Masters Degree in Advanced Clinical Practice in Primary Care. Her provisional conclusions from her experiences and study were that the role of nurse as alternative first point of contact probably worked better in smaller practices, a theoretical background and training in pharmacology were essential to the nurse practitioner role, and she was increasingly unclear where nurses in general practice were heading, although specialisation may spell part of the answer.

Conclusions

What are the lessons from the Derbyshire project and other evaluations of the nurse practitioner movement in the UK? The first contentious issue is that of training and recognition. Until the UKCC spells out the role, function, prescribing rights and training requirements of nurse practitioners, they will always be in a kind of professional limbo, despite the availability of the various Diploma and Masters courses. In the meantime, it has to be recognised that a mix of practice-based mentorships, mirrored consultations, one-to-one tutorials, as well as external course attendance is the way forward because of the requirement to bring medical colleagues on board and keep them on board. The experience of the nurses in the Derbyshire project suggests that attending higher level courses teaches not only advanced clinical expertise, but also a greater assertiveness which allows nurses to take their place alongside, rather than as assistants to, family doctors.

This brings us to the second issue: the notion of putting an end to the employer–employee relationship and going for full partnership, which was raised at the time of the project and during the update interviews, although it did not surface as a burning concern. Some of the doctors and one of the nurses were very keen, although the current remuneration arrangements in primary care (*The Red Book*) were perceived as a major barrier. The Primary Care Act of 1997 has removed the regulatory barrier, but there has been no flood of applications. Just as some doctors are shying away from the lifelong commitment of a partnership, many nurses may not be ready to exchange the flexibility of the staff position for the financial responsibility of a partnership. There are also undoubtedly cultural influences at work. How many nurses went into the profession with this end in mind? Over the past ten years, new professional and financial structures, from *The Scope of Professional Practice* (UKCC, 1992), nurse prescribing, to the Primary Care Act (1997) have been put in place, but until there is a critical mass of nurses willing to exploit the new professional as well as clinical freedoms, progress towards nurse partnerships is likely to be slow.

The final issue relates to nurses in the management of the new NHS. Since April 1999, PCGs have been responsible for addressing health needs in their local populations, improving the quality of primary care and commissioning specialist care for their patients. The majority on the boards of PCGs are GPs (seven) with only two nurses to provide the nursing contribution. It is going to be a tall order to get the nursing voice heard; the positive signs from the nurse practitioner experience are that nurses may, through autonomous practice and working alongside medical colleagues, feel more confident in contributing to rather than reacting to the health management agenda, and thus be ready to play a full part when a more sensible board configuration and management structure emerge with the moves towards Primary Care Trusts.

References

Balint E *et al.* (1993) *The Doctor, the Patient and the Group.* Routledge, London.

Bowling A (1981) *Delegation in General Practice: A Study of Doctors and Nurses.* Tavistock, London.

Campbell S (1997) Nurse practitioners at the cutting edge of today's NHS. *Primary Care* 7(8): 2–4.

Chambers N (1995) Report on a study to obtain a patients' and carers' perspective of the nursing services provided by the Darley Dale primary health care team. Unpublished.

Chambers N (1996) *Nurse practitioners in primary care: an alternative to a consultation with the doctor?* PhD thesis, University of Manchester.

Chambers N (1998) *Nurse Practitioners in Primary Care.* Radcliffe Medical Press, Oxford.

Coopers and Lybrand (1996) *Nurse Practitioner Evaluation Project.* Coopers and Lybrand, Uxbridge, Middlesex.

Crail M (1998) Price of new doctors may be change in role. *Health Service Journal* **30 July**: 8.

Greenwood L (1998) Direct action. *NHS Magazine* **Summer**: 11.

Holmes G *et al.* (1976) Contribution of a nurse clinician to office practice productivity. *Health Services Research* **II** (I): 1–33.

Johnson W (1997) The nurse practitioner in primary care. *Primary Care* **7**(4): 10–12.

Kaufman G (1996) Nurse practitioners in general practice: an expanding role. *Nursing Standard* **11**(8): 44–7.

Miles A (1991) *Women, Health and Medicine.* Open University Press, Milton Keynes.

Office of Health Technology Assessment (1986) *Nurse Practitioners: A Policy Analysis Health Technology Case Study No 37.* Washington DC, USA.

Poulton B (1995) Keeping the customer satisfied. *Primary Health Care* **5**(4): 16–19.

Robinson G, Beaton S and White P (1993) Attitudes towards practice nurses: a survey of a sample of general practitioners in England and Wales. *British Journal of General Practice* **43**: 25–9.

Stilwell B (1988) Nurse practitioners in British general practice. In: A Bowling and B Stilwell (eds) *The Nurse in Family Practice.* Scutari, London.

Stilwell B (1991) An ideal consultation. In: J Salvage (ed) *Nurse Practitioners: Working for Change in Primary Health Care Nursing.* Kings Fund, London.

Touche Ross (1994) *Evaluation of Nurse Practitioners Pilot Projects.* Touche Ross, London.

UKCC (1992) *The Scope of Professional Practice.* United Kingdom Central Council for Nursing, Midwifery and Health Visiting, London.

CHAPTER FOUR

Serving the community: a nurse-led minor injuries service

Margaret Bamford

> *only one in ten patients attending these departments required referral to a specialist or return visit to the department, the remaining nine were discharged home, or into the care of their own GP.* (Audit Commission, 1996)

The service and its context

With difficulties being experienced in the NHS through staff shortages in medical specialities, changes in primary care service delivery and increasing expectations of the public, the pressures on Accident and Emergency (A&E) departments have never been greater. Doctors, and therefore medical skills, are in particularly short supply. This chapter reports on a study designed to meet the skill deficit and the public's need for a safe, efficient and effective A&E service by provision of specially trained nurses as the first point of contact. The study was funded by the NHS West Midlands Research and Development Directorate, and was completed in June 1998 (Bamford *et al.*, 1998).

There is a requirement to reduce the hours that junior doctors work (DoH, 1990), and in some instances junior doctors have been withdrawn from A&E departments because of training difficulties, such as lack of supervision and exposure to a sufficient range of experience (Garnett and Elton, 1991). Reduction in junior doctors' hours is one of a string of events which leads managers to consider substitution or alternative provision of service (Cavanagh and Bamford, 1997). This service crisis is set to increase. Within the next ten to 15 years there is going to be a major shortage of doctors. Some specialist areas will be harder hit than others, including general practice and primary care, psychiatry, and A&E services. In 1999 the UK government invited proposals from the higher education sector for universities to extend existing medical school provision. Against this backdrop nurses, midwives and health visitors are changing and extending their working practices: not only in those areas in which junior doctors work. It would be misleading to see their development as just a solution to a particular resource problem. The issues underpinning role development of professional groups are much wider and are driven by a combination of service needs and the provision of efficient, effective, clinically competent health service professionals to address them. Increasingly, traditional roles and practices will give way to more flexible and collaborative ways of working.

The nurse-led minor injuries unit (NLMIU)

Some A&E departments are establishing new NLMIUs and GP-led primary care units within their existing facilities to deal with the range and breadth of public demand. Some NLMIUs are, however, well established, such as the one described in this study.

The community hospital where the research was carried out is quite large, with 124 beds. The emphasis is on rehabilitation and care of the elderly. The casualty department has been available to the local community in one form or another for many years, and is an important element and focus for healthcare for this population. The area is rural, with horticulture and agriculture the main occupations and many people commuting to the nearby larger cities for their work.

The casualty department 'sees' about 12 000 patients a year. Nearly 60% of these patients are seen, diagnosed, treated and discharged by the nurses working in the department. There are 7.5 members of nursing staff in the NLMIU at the community hospital, providing a 24-hour, 7-day per week service. Local GPs are available for advice and consultation about their own particular patients. An 'out-of-hours' primary care service is provided by local doctors from 6pm until 8am. People who are able to travel to the casualty department are encouraged to do so, and doctors go out on call from the casualty department during this time. There is an agreement with the local ambulance service that only appropriate patients will be brought to the casualty department, but sometimes people arrive by car with relatives, and then have to be transferred to the local A&E department about 17 miles away.

A working definition of a nurse-led minor injuries service was designed for the research project (Bamford *et al.*, 1998). This was:

> *A nurse-led minor injuries service is a service to a community, led and managed by nurses, to offer appropriate care for minor conditions, illness and injury, which would not be expected to be treated by an accident and emergency department, and for which the patient would not normally attend a GP service.*

Range of methods used in the project

A range of methods was used to collect data. These were:

- a focus group activity using the Nominal Group Technique (NGT) was held with lead nurses in NLMIU in the West Midlands to identify current activity (*n* = 9)
- a scoping exercise of all services in the West Midlands Region describing themselves as NLMIU (ten units were found which matched the definition)
- a six-month snapshot of activity in a longstanding NLMIU within the West Midlands (6196 potential records existed)
- a 'case-matching' exercise with a large A&E inner-city department managed by consultants (414 cases were identified for matching)
- a survey of the perceived education and training needs of nurses working in NLMIU in the West Midlands Region (*n* = 106) (Wilkes, 1997)
- a survey of nurses' perceived information needs in a large A&E department in an Acute Trust and two NLMIU in a Community Trust (*n* = 17) (Pope, 1997)
- a survey of patients' and users' perceptions of a local NLMIU (*n* = 400)
- a review by an expert panel of outcomes of treatment in a NLMIU (*n* = 414 records).

The NGT is perhaps the one method in this list of which readers may not have heard. It is a consensus decision-making process, using a focus group approach with a panel of experts. The technique was developed by Van de Ven and Delbecq (1974) in the 1960s and early 1970s, initially on the NASA space programme, when difficult and complex issues needed to be decided. The process is fairly structured for a focus group, but when expert time is used, it is at a premium. (For more information on the process see Van de Ven and Delbecq, 1972 and 1974.)

Findings

Range and type of service

Attendees are shown by diagnostic group in Table 4.1.

The largest number of attendances at the NLMIU during the six-month period under analysis was for people with lacerations (1127; 18%). Of these 65% were dealt with wholly by the nurses in the department. In 18% of instances the doctor was called for advice or to be given information about the patient. In reality this usually constituted arrangements for issuing antibiotics (which in the UK requires a doctor's prescription). Only 17% of this group had conditions that

Table 4.1:   Diagnostic groups

All attendees 1/7/96–22/12/96	
Lacerations	1127 (18%)
Other	909 (15%)
Other diagnosis, including non-specified	584 (9%)
Joint injury	404 (7%)
Other medical	348 (6%)
Foreign body	334 (5%)
Respiratory	239 (4%)
Muscle/tendon	221 (4%)
Bite/sting	215 (3%)
Abrasions	209 (3%)
Fractures	208 (3%)
Sprains/ligaments	206 (3%)
Concussion	204 (3%)
ENT	194 (3%)
Contusion	187 (3%)
Local sepsis	178 (3%)
Other head injury	157 (3%)
Abdominal pain	165 (3%)
Burn/scald	107 (2%)
	6196 (100%)

were sufficiently severe to necessitate subsequently being seen by the patient's GP.

The next largest group of patients were categorised as 'other' (909, 15%). Unfortunately this classification does not give a clear indication of this group of patients' needs. This is because, at this time, the form used in the casualty department had been designed to support a local public health accident prevention scheme rather than the work of the department.

The largest group of patients that the nurses called the doctor in to see was 'abdominal pain' (n=165), 85% of that group. The next highest group was 'respiratory' (n= 239) with 78%. The next two highest categories for doctor referral were 'ENT' (n=194), 73%, and 'other medical' (n=348), 71%.

Table 4.2 indicates that the only diagnoses where a GP was not called – over half of the occasions – were patients with a burn or a scald (84%), a laceration (65%) and a sprain or ligament damage (52%).

The largest diagnostic groups that the nurses dealt with in their entirety were 'burns/scalds' (n=107) at 84%, 'lacerations' (n=1127) at 65%, and 'sprains and ligaments' (n=206) at 52% of all cases. The group of patients who were classified as 'GP called for advice/information' were a difficult group to classify. When this group of patients were discussed with the nurses, it became clear that the patients fell into areas of treatment which at that time could not be dealt with totally by the nurses because of policy or statutory limitations. These included prescribing authority, or the referral authority to request further investigations within the NHS.

In all the records reviewed (n=6196), 37% of presenting patients were seen and dealt with totally by the nurses, 21% fell into the grey area of 'GP called for advice/information' (which in probability still meant that the nurses dealt with the patient), and those who saw their GP, which was 42%.

The advice/information category is confusing. What happens in reality is that the nurse will still deal with and manage the totality of the patient experience. However, in some circumstances the nurse will inform the patient's GP of the course of action that is being taken (it may be a day or two before the patient goes to see his/her GP). In other circumstances, the nurse will contact the GP for advice, particularly if it is felt that the patient will need a course of antibiotics. In these circumstances the patient will often be fitted into a GP session that day to be given a prescription.

Table 4.2: Most common diagnoses* by contact with GP/doctor

Diagnosis	GP not called	GP called for advice/ information	Saw doctor**
Abdominal pain (n=165)	4%	13%	83%
Abrasion (n=209)	47%	23%	30%
Bite/sting (n=215)	45%	23%	32%
Burn/scald (n=107)	84%	8%	8%
Concussion (n=204)	42%	20%	38%
Contusion (n=187)	41%	27%	32%
ENT (n=194)	7%	20%	73%
Foreign body (n=334)	33%	28%	39%
Fracture (n=208)	27%	26%	47%
Joint injury (n=404)	45%	18%	37%
Laceration (n=1127)	65%	18%	17%
Local sepsis (n=178)	21%	19%	60%
Muscle/tendon (n=221)	47%	20%	33%
Defined 'other' (n=909)	32%	21%	47%
Other head injury (n=157)	22%	40%	37%
Other medical (n=348)	10%	20%	71%
Respiratory (n=239)	5%	17%	78%
Sprain/ligament (n=206)	52%	18%	30%
Other diagnoses (including 'non-specified') (n=584)	23%	25%	52%
Total (n=6196)	37%	21%	42%

*A doctor saw all 21 cardiac patients and advised or saw 35 out of 36 of the patients with central nervous system damage, 19 of the 23 patients with a dislocation, 35 out of 39 patients with an infectious disease and all four psychiatric patients.
**Saw doctor includes: GP called to attend, doctor in department, and seen by duty doctor at surgery.

Delivering service and service outcomes

In the study, 'outcome' means the end point of the visit. This may not of course be the end of the care episode for the patient. A more severe patient arriving at the NLMIU would be immediately transferred to the local A&E department.

This part of the study was designed to evaluate differences in outcome between the NLMI unit and a large, inner city A&E department run in a traditional (medically managed) way. The aim was to see if there were any major differences in outcome for particular categories of patient visit. It could be anticipated, for example, that there would be cost differences, the infrastructure and personnel costs in an A&E

department being higher. If there were no differences in outcome, however, for a similar group of (NLMI) patients it raises the question, why are patients not dealt with differently in an A&E department? One explanation which could be given is that of the cost of building and supporting medical hegemony. The building and establishing of junior doctors' education and their clinical decision making is expensive and time consuming. It might be asked why medical consultations are universally required as a norm in A&E departments. Is it justified asking some non-urgent patients to wait for four hours (and maybe longer) for a medical consultation? Can a nurse meet their needs more efficiently and as effectively?

For this part of the evaluation, 6196 case notes were randomly withdrawn from the community hospital archives for the six months from July to December 1996. Staff within the casualty department did this work. These case notes were anonomised, the information available to the researchers was: patient number; age; sex; date of visit; post (zip) code; occupation; time of visit; initial diagnosis or presenting condition; nursing assessment, treatment and outcome. These notes provided the basic information for the researchers, and from this base 450 records were randomly withdrawn. Only 414 of these records were subsequently able to be used.

These 414 records were then matched with similar records from the large A&E department in an inner-city hospital. The records were matched for age, sex and presenting condition. Although the request to the A&E department was for a similar number of records, in the event, 135 records did not have a match, leaving only 279 records which could be compared for outcome (*see* Table 4.3).

Although 279 records is not a large volume of records for analysis, it is sufficient to be an indicator. Of these analysed records the results indicated that the same outcome occurred in 165 (59%) instances. That is, the same outcome if the person was cared for in the NLMI unit or the high technology (medically managed) A&E department. This leads to

Table 4.3: Analysis of matched records

Category	Number	Percentage
	(n=279)	(100)
Same outcome	165	59
Different outcome	85	30.5
Patient left department without treatment	18	6.5
Problem with the record	11	4

the conclusion that many minor illness and injuries can be dealt with by experienced and well-prepared nurses.

A different outcome (85 patients, 31%) occurred for a range of reasons between the A&E unit and the NLMIU. One reason was that from the information available in the A&E daybook it was very difficult to match cases; description of injuries was not clear. Local 'shorthand' was used, and when the records were analysed the conditions did not match. Often this was because of the severity of the patients condition attending the A&E department. This finding only serves to highlight (yet again) the importance of use of common codes for describing conditions, and good information systems to support practitioners in their work environment. If we do not have systems that speak to one another it will be impossible to analyse what is being done across services, and subsequently make it much more difficult to track and evaluate the practice of professionals and so change and advance service delivery.

Implications for nursing and service delivery

The following research questions were addressed in the study and will be used to explore the policy in practice issues identified in the results.

1   Do NLMIU provide a service to the community which is at least equal to a similar type of service provided by other professionals or mix of professionals?

A   It seems that they do. The public understand, accept and value the NLMI service. Managers and professionals are confused, however. There is a lack of clarity in the definition, interpretation and implementation of the role of the nurse in this area of immediate care and this leads to confusion for some health professionals and purchasers of healthcare.

Where there is some concern about nurses expanding their role into less traditional areas of care, lack of role clarity could be both an enabler and a restrictor to practice development. Until very recently adoption of (previously) 'medical' skills has been viewed quite negatively both within the nursing profession and outside of it. If more research was carried out into comparative care outcomes this position might change and the value of expanded roles for nurses be realised. Additionally, adequate role definition and preparation is particularly important now in the UK because of the increased emphasis on clinical governance and the legal position of the practitioner in providing care (NHSE, 1998).

B There needs to be clear role preparation and educational opportunity for nurses (and probably other professionals) working in this area of care. Current preparation for this role is not nationally specified, and provision of opportunity is limited. The opportunities for multidisciplinary education and training are also limited, this compounds prejudices about who can provide what care and is antithetical to teamworking and partnership in care; the proposed direction for the new NHS (Labour government reforms).

C There should be a review of the role and contribution of community hospitals in relation to their contribution to health gain in a locality. Many such units are closing, regarded as unsafe and uneconomical. Perhaps there is a need to think of their contribution differently, particularly in rural areas.

D The consultation document on prescribing (DoH, 1999) presents an opportunity for nurses working in NLMIU to make clear their prescribing arrangements. They need to be able to safely treat a larger proportion of minor injuries and illnesses that are occurring in their locality. Again, there will be education and training needs attached to this activity.

E There needs to be a robust 'risk management' exercise to identify potential areas of risk for practitioners which can then be addressed by appropriate education and training.

F There needs to be improvement in the recording of information. This is important for both organisational and professional reasons.

2 Do NLMIU provide a service to the community which would otherwise be unmet?

A Some people come to the NLMIU just for advice and reassurance, and it may be that this role will be subsumed within the remit of NHS Direct (nurse-run telephone health advice service) when it 'rolls out' from the current pilot sites. There is, however, an excellent opportunity for health promotion, not only in relation to current health need, but also on wider health concerns within a community. It will probably require more extensive education and training for nurses working in NLMIU if they are to maximise their influence with patients and carers.

B NLMIU are able to offer a quick-response service to individuals, and to provide reassurance. This will encourage people to get things 'checked out' rather than leaving them untreated.

C There does not seem to be an issue in most people's minds about whether they are seen by a doctor or a nurse. They just want to be seen by someone and have their problem dealt with. They trusted the nurse to refer them to a doctor if it was thought necessary.

D Patients themselves appear to be making decisions about the severity of their conditions and seeking appropriate help. With more focused patient/population education this element of self-care could be enhanced.

3 Are NLMIU an acceptable provider of care for people?

A Overwhelmingly patients and users like this service. This is evident in the numbers of people who use the service and parents who bring their children for care.

B The relatively low referral rate for further treatment is suggestive of a good understanding of the role and uses of casualty by the respondents, and of the effectiveness of the department. Further work could be undertaken to identify patients using the neighbouring A&E departments and their reasons for doing so.

C Inter-professional issues may interfere in the delivery of this type of service. What is offered is a nursing service which facilitates access to a medical service, where this is necessary. Not all the problems dealt with in the NLMIU are medical, or in some cases even nursing. The professional issues here are those around prescribing, supervision of practice and adoption of practices which may previously have been seen as the work of a medical practitioner. Additionally the range of 'problems' that people present with and which may appear at one level to be a health issue may subsequently be revealed to be social, or related to equity or deprivation issues.

Given this complexity it would be a mistake to compare the service in an NLMIU with a medical service in every aspect, but measurement of outcomes for similar medical conditions could be a good place to start.

4 Can a NLMIU provide a safe level of care and service to a community?

A Public acceptance is a good indicator of a perceived safe service – people in a community would not keep attending if there was an indication that the service was not safe. The number of children brought to the casualty by their parents (in this study, 25% of departmental work) is a good subjective measure of perceptions of safety.

B From the work done in comparing records for outcomes and expert panel views, it would seem that the service is safe. Fundamental to any concept of safety, however, is the preparation of the people who deliver the service to a population, and the support they are given by the organisation which employs them. Continuing education is a cause for concern (*see* **E** below).

C All but one of the units in the main study had protocols for practice, the majority of which were the result of joint development between medical and nursing staff. This endorses the view of Duff *et al.* (1996) in relation to the benefits of ownership and communication of protocols and guidelines. Some protocols in this survey were not adopted from national guidelines, however, and this raises concerns regarding the extent of underpinning research and the consistency of standards of care (Tingle and Cribb, 1996). There is a need to develop common standards and protocols for this area of care. Evidence-based practice should be the cornerstone for these developments.

D Qualitative data regarding the use of protocols in practice also offer some inconsistencies in the findings. Whilst the main theme to emerge was the view that protocols provide an opportunity to ensure that an acceptable level of quality care is delivered, there was evidence to suggest that staff also believed protocols provide a legal framework which safeguards their practice. Austin and Herbert (1995) point to this issue with concern, claiming staff may be encouraged to undertake roles and responsibilities beyond their level of experience under the misapprehension that, if they follow the directions exactly, they will be protected.

E A substantial number of staff currently employed within minor injuries units has already achieved diploma and degree status. This trend is set to continue with all pre-registration programmes awarding a diploma in higher education alongside the professional qualification. A disproportionate number of staff had undertaken the Emergency Nurse

Practitioner course and the findings confirmed those of Dolan *et al.* (1997) who highlighted the lack of standardisation within these courses and a mismatch of content with the learning needs of nurses working within nurse-led minor injuries services. This links back to the constant thread through this research, around role clarity and preparation, and managing risk. It implies that the statuatory nursing body, the UKCC, should be interested in this area of service provision, in their role of safeguarding the public.

F The majority of staff believed that nurses did need to undertake a recognised course to enable them to work in minor injuries, many clearly describing their area as a specialised field. They reinforce the need to not only address the specific clinical subjects relating to the types of minor injuries, but also the wider context within which their practice is based, such as medico-legal issues and implications of autonomous decision making.

G The information needs of these nurses are diverse, as are the methods they employ to fulfil those needs. Indications are that immediacy and convenience are the keys to the sources chosen, and information need dictates the final resource selection. For research purposes, course work and general enquiry interviewees were more likely to consult journals or go to the library. For clinical decision making and practice of the role in general, more immediate information is gathered from sources on hand; colleagues, sales representatives from medical supplies companies or personal collections.

H Questions are raised as to why certain sources are used more than others and this indicates that there are barriers to obtaining information from the various sources. During their working day, nurses are busy within their units and have little time to access information. There is also a lack of resources at hospital sites, which means that the need for immediate or convenient information is not being met.

I Managers need to address nurses' continuing education needs. Managers of services need to ensure that practitioners, of all groups, are fit for practice and fit for purpose. Because of the way that NLMIU have developed these issues will need to be addressed at both a personal and organisational level. There will need to be appropriate systems in place to support safe working practices. These include:

• policy development to support practice
• development of minimum standards for education and training to support practice

- clear service specifications to clarify type and range of service
- information systems which describe type and range of decision making
- information systems and documentation to support evidence-based practice.

Lack of information systems to support practice is a potential area of risk for patient safety. Practitioners seem to be dependent on inappropriate sources of 'evidence' to support their decision making. Persuading all healthcare practitioners that they need to put personal effort into continuing professional education is difficult (Sackett *et al.*, 1997). It is even more difficult if it is a constant 'unequal struggle' amongst a range of competing demands, i.e. work, home and family. There has to be a way of making this task easier, and managers, as well as individual practitioners, should take responsibility for updating.

Conclusions: advancing and extending nursing practice

This research study has shown that many minor illness and injury episodes can be dealt with successfully by experienced and well-prepared nurses. Additionally, whether they are 'seen' by a doctor or a nurse is not an issue for most people. They just want to be seen by someone and have their problem dealt with. They trust a nurse to refer them to a doctor if s/he thinks it is necessary.

Nurses working in NLMIUs need legislative assistance in order to more fully achieve their potential. There is likely to be contention about role change. Any activity which challenges long-held views has the potential for causing concern. Some medical colleagues feel that only a doctor can do some things, they think that other professional groups taking on a wider role can only be detrimental. An example of this is the development of nurse prescribing. District nurses and health visitors in the UK can prescribe from a very restricted list of products, none of which would be considered a major risk to patients; many of the items on the list are dressings and very simple medicines (DoH, 1989; UK, 1992; UK, 1994). The concern is probably less about competency, but more about role substitution (nurse versus doctor) issues (Cavanagh and Bamford, 1997). There are hopeful signs of change, however. The Crown Report (DoH, 1999) suggests that prescribing rights be extended to include a wider range of health professionals.

Initial treatment for minor injuries is an area of nursing practice that is seen as successful and growing. Nurses are involved in offering initial treatment for minor injuries in the community (Bowles, 1993; Marsh and Dawes, 1995), in the workplace (McEwen *et al.*, 1979; Bamford, 1993), and in both A&E units and minor injuries units (Garnett and Elton, 1991; Dale *et al.*, 1994; Kilshaw, 1994; Newman, 1994; Brown, 1995).

Amongst recent studies of the NHS is a review of A&E services in England and Wales (Audit Commission, 1996). Researchers found that only one in ten patients attending these departments required referral to a specialist or a return visit to the department, the remaining nine were discharged home or into the care of their own GP, with less than 0.5% attending with conditions considered to be life-threatening. Amongst the recommendations of the Audit Commission is the development of programmes of specific education for nurses, endorsed by the regulatory bodies for nurse education. This, it is believed, will enable nurses to expand their range of skills and play a more active role in the treatment of minor injuries and illness.

Current programmes available for nurses working in NLMIU are focused on locally perceived need, are usually of two to three weeks duration and concern skill acquisition (Keltie, 1993). When thinking about the range and depth of work that nurses do in NLMI units it is obvious that current forms of preparation are inadequate. Nurses working in these complex settings have very specific education and training needs. These range from problem identification, physical examination, questioning, analysis and synthesis of information, decision making, diagnosis, information giving and teaching, treatment and discharge, and, at some time in the future, prescribing of medicines.

These skills and knowledge are not acquired over a short timespan, or by experience. Nurses need to learn, to be coached, to be tested and to gain confidence in a safe environment if they are to be of real benefit to a community and make a contribution to health gain. There needs to be an acknowledgement of the need for this specific education and training, which should be to a national standard and fit into a standard post-registration programme, carrying higher education accreditation.

One final point worth noting is that the more that research into these non-traditional areas of care is done, the clearer the need and supply picture will be. Better education, management and practice strategies can then be devised to serve and safeguard the public.

References

Audit Commission (1996) *By Accident or Design: Improving A&E Services in England and Wales*. HMSO, London.

Austin C and Herbert I (1995) Clinical guidelines: should we be worried? *British Journal of Occupational Therapy* **58**(11): 481–4.

Bamford M (1993) *Aspects of Health Among an Employed Population*. Doctoral thesis, The University of Aston, Birmingham.

Bamford M, Wilkes J, Pope A, Edwards A, Jordan K and Warder J (1998) *Nurse-led Minor Injuries Services: An Evaluative Study into Nursing Interventions*. Centre for Health Planning and Management, Keele University.

Bowles A (1993) Negotiating the change: from practice nurse to nurse practitioner. *Nurse Practitioners: The UK/USA Experience*, First International Conference on Nurse Practitioner Practice, Nursing Standard/RCN, London, 6–8 August.

Brown P (1995) Minor injuries, major advance. *Nursing Management* **2**(2): 8–9.

Cavanagh SJ and Bamford M (1997) Substitution in nursing practice: clinical, management and research implications. *Journal of Nursing Management* **5**(6): 333–9.

Dale J, Dolan B and Lang H (1994) *Health Care in Folkestone and Deal: New Directions for the Minor Injuries Units*. King's A&E Primary Care Service and Kent Family Health Services Authority.

DoH (1989) *Report of the Advisory Group on Nurse Prescribing*. Department of Health, London.

DoH (1990) *Heads of Agreement. Ministerial Group on Junior Doctor's Hours*. Department of Health, London.

DoH (1999) *Review of Prescribing, Supply and Administration of Medicines*. Department of Health, London.

Dolan B, Dale J and Morley V (1997) Nurse practitioners: the role in A&E and primary care. *Nursing Standard* **11**(17): 33–8.

Duff L, Kitson A, Seers K and Humphries D (1996) Clinical guidelines: an introduction to their development and implementation. *Journal of Advanced Nursing* **23**: 887–95.

Garnett SM and Elton PJ (1991) A treatment service for minor injuries: maintaining equity of access. *Journal of Public Health Medicine* **13**(4): 260–6.

Keltie D (1993) Emergency nurse practitioners: the Derby Way. *Nurse Practitioners: The UK/USA Experience*. First International Conference on Nurse Practitioner Practice, Nursing Standard/RCN, London, 6–8 August.

Kilshaw LE (1994) *Workplace accidents at a community hospital casualty unit*. Unpublished report, University of Birmingham.

Marsh GN and Dawes ML (1995) Establishing a minor illness nurse in a busy general practice. *BMJ* **310**: 778–80.

McEwen J, Pearson JCG and Langham A (1979) *Report to the Health and Safety Executive: Treatment of Injuries and Emergencies Arising at Work.* Department of Community Health, University of Nottingham.

NHSE (1998) *A First-Class Service.* National Health Service Executive, London.

Newman P (1994) *Evaluation of the St. Albans Minor Injury Unit.* Dept. of Public Health Medicine, NW Thames Regional Health Authority.

Pope A (1997) *Information needs and information provision for nurses practising in the NLMIU and an A&E department in light of research-based practice.* Unpublished dissertation, University of Central England, Birmingham.

Sackett DL, Scott Richardson W, Rosenberg W and Haynes RB (1997) *Evidence-based Medicine: How to Practice and Teach EBM.* Churchill Livingstone, London.

Tingle J and Cribb A (1996) *Nursing Law and Ethics.* Blackwell Science, Oxford.

UK (1992) *Medicinal Products: Prescription by Nurses etc. Act 1992.* HMSO, London.

UK (1994) *Medicinal Products: Prescription by Nurses etc. Act (Commencement No. 1) Order 1994.* HMSO, London.

Van de Ven AH and Delbecq AL (1974) The effectiveness of Nominal, Delphi and interacting group decision-making processes. *Academy of Management Journal* **17**(4): 605–21.

Wilkes J (1997) *Exploring the nurse's role within nurse-led minor injuries services and their perceived development needs to enable them to practice effectively.* Unpublished dissertation, University of Warwick.

The United States

Healthcare, health policy and nursing

Rosemary Goodyear

Healthcare in the United States has progressed from folklore healing practices to far-reaching technological advancements in a little over a century. Traversing through the belief systems of illness as a punishment and quackery cures to scientific medicine was similar around the globe. However, it was not until early in this century that a solid foundation for a scientific framework was established. Education of physicians in Europe, epidemics, wars and the capabilities of surgical intervention served as markers and forums for the current healthcare system in the US.

The foundation for scientific medicine was marked through the establishment of university education for physicians, the transitioning of hospitals from almshouses to places of care and the initiation of nursing as a profession. The hospitals quickly found the nurse to be an inexpensive source of help. The number of nursing schools grew from three in 1873 to 432 by 1900 to 1129 by 1910.

The healthcare market

The healthcare market grew from the hospital sector. The growth and success of hospital services was due, in a large part, to the introduction of surgical procedures. The physician's home/office was no longer acceptable for these procedures and interventions; wealthy patients were more accepting of these services when they were provided in hospitals specifically designed for this type of care. Support by the upper classes prompted the building and financing of specialty hospitals. By the early 20th century, private hospitals came under financial exigency and their administrators selected the only other alternative available to bureaucratic organisations to meet expenses: patient fees were raised to cover costs. This method greatly increased the income of the hospitals and, as a result, began to alter the healthcare landscape. It was in 1922 that the New York Academy of Medicine reported that hospitals were recording budget surpluses. The healthcare marketplace had its beginning with this action.

The country's progress through financial booms, a depression, and the introduction of health insurance also marked this era of change. Health insurance for the individual came about in the 1930s and altered the existing method of generating income for hospitals. The introduction of a risk-free health plan for a monthly fee likewise changed healthcare practice in the US from a service to an industry. Around the world governments were beginning to institute healthcare programmes for all citizens residing in their countries. The US, on the other hand, elected to initiate the private insurance model, which supported the country's ideology of individualism and capitalism. This approach was reinforced in the confrontation between the physicians and the government when a plan for health coverage for the poor was written into the Social Security Act of 1935. The legislation mentioned mandatory health insurance and this was fiercely opposed by the American Medical Association (AMA). The bill had to be amended and the section stipulating care of the poor removed so that the original policy would pass in Congress (government). This was a demonstration of the power of the AMA at that time and little has changed through the decades. The AMA continues to be one of the largest contributors of funds toward the election and re-election of representatives to Congress, the policy-making body in the US (Starr, 1982).

Managed care

The concept of managed care was not new to the delivery of health services in the US, but its resurgence in the 1990s was seen as a possible solution worth revisiting. In the 1930s the economic advantages of a healthy workforce were recognised by business. Physician practices to promote and maintain health were provided and were successful in company towns. Kaiser, a corporation contracted to build a dam in the western part of the US, hired physicians to keep the workers healthy so that the dam could be built on schedule. These workers and families had been relocated to the construction site; away from all normal consumer resources, including healthcare.

From its earliest form, managed care has held the concept of health maintenance as a primary goal. The introduction of a variety of new models focusing on fiscal constraints and improving cost-effectiveness are present in today's models. Economists, social policy makers, insurance companies, government and the corporate world all submitted their ideas and potential solutions to the problem. The political fury over the Health Security Act proposed by the Clinton administration in 1993 was a demonstration of what has been said to be an over-ambitious attempt for a complete overhaul of the healthcare system, while the consumer only wanted a quick fix and reduced costs. Two Pulitzer Prize-winning journalists, Johnson and Broder (1996), comment that the issue that influenced the rejection of this reform proposal was not the policy, but a society who:

> . . . was less fair in dealing with its poor, its ill and its disabled.

Anderson *et al.* (1996) indicate that the failure of comprehensive healthcare reform did not make the problems go away, but instead clarified them. First the industry had to deal with the issue incrementally, rather than in a comprehensive form; second there would have to be greater reliance on the marketplace, rather than government regulation.

Managed care, a corporate model for delivering healthcare, is currently being phased in throughout the US. Some states are far advanced in accomplishing this task while other sections of the country are moving more slowly and observing at a distance. The insurance industry is in control of designing and establishing programmes to cover their consumers, with the goal of delivering quality and comprehensive services at a reduced cost. Many of the initial managed care companies no longer exist, due to insolvency or mergers (market forces). Programmes that work in one state may not work in other states. For this reason, state governments were given a great deal of latitude to create programmes that would fit their population and resources. Managed Care Organisations (MCOs) would then bid on contracts to implement these programmes. A fact that has emerged from successes and failures of these companies is that a critical mass of people in a concentrated geographic area is needed to produce positive results. The managed care programmes for the Medicaid populations, an assistance programme, and Medicare, an eligibility programme for the aged, are two examples of federally funded healthcare. Both programmes are managed by private insurance companies such as Blue Cross and Blue Shield. In essence, the federal or state government contracts with these insurance companies to administer their programmes. These companies contract, on a state-by-state basis, to develop and implement managed care programmes for those enrolled. The companies must meet federal and state guidelines in order to develop and administer these MCO programmes. In addition they may operate private and/or corporate contracts in each state.

The funding of healthcare in the US is essentially divided into three segments. One third of the funds are contributed by the federal government, one third through the corporate insurance market and one third by the individual patient or fee for service. Inequalities in coverage exist. With the introduction of MCOs in 1993 the statistics in 1996 demonstrated that Texas had 24% of their population uninsured, while Wisconsin had only 8.4% uninsured.

Public health services

Concurrent with the rise of medicine in hospitals and nurse training in hospitals, the field of public health emerged. It was the protection of the public's health from disease that directed its focus to sanitation and engineering rather than medicine. In the mid-19th century, state governments began to develop departments of health. The first successful state board to monitor the public's health was in Massachusetts. Their activities centred on monitoring the occupations of commerce, transport and the quarantine of ships found to be carrying disease. Another focus was centred on the tenements in the large seaport communities where the masses of immigrants lived. It was at this time that the role of the public health nurse was initiated.

The scientific ability to identify the source of infection strengthened public health's alliance with medicine. It was the view of the private physician that the treatment of diseases such as tuberculosis and venereal disease was within their scope of practice and that public health was intruding into their practice. Likewise, the public dispensary that provided medicines to the poor for free was attacked by the medical community as another method of depriving the physician of an income. The situation was reported (Anderson *et al.*, 1998) that:

> *Vast sums of money are wasted yearly on worthless and undeserving persons.*

The public dispensaries were eventually absorbed into the medical schools in the mid-1920s. These became the sites where the medical interns gained experience, but patients were also charged for the services. Public health was also classified as municipal socialism and unfair competition with the physician in private practice. Health services in schools were another area that physicians cited as unfair competition and therefore children had to be sent home to be treated by the private physicians. Thus the detection and referral of illness became the only programme permitted in public schools by physicians in the service of public health. Early in the 20th century disease prevention through healthy living, the establishment of paediatrics with a focus on prevention, the fight against tuberculosis, and increasing demand for pre-employment physicals changed the face of the discipline.

Today the illness profile of the population is not dissimilar to that of the UK. Western diseases (cancers, coronary heart disease, strokes, hypertension and obesity) combined account for most disease morbidity, and health inequalities in terms of ethnicity, gender, class and locality exist. In the US, however, inequalities are compounded by the lack of universal healthcare coverage referred to above. Currently in the US there are around 43 million people who are uninsured for healthcare.

Additionally (see Chapter Six), the US has witnessed a growing emergence of complex health and social problems. Teen pregnancy, HIV and AIDS, substance use, domestic and gang-related violence, a growing elderly population, and demographic shifts of diverse populations challenge the way healthcare is defined, and where and how it is provided. While healthcare has typically been delivered in expensive, acute-care hospital settings, the effort to contain costs in today's managed care system has meant a dramatic shift towards providing care in co-ordinated and less-expensive community and ambulatory care settings.

Nursing

The origins of today's healthcare delivery system in the US can be found in the review of the history of medicine, hospitals and public health. However, no discipline would be where it is today without the discipline of nursing. Medicine would not have reliable colleagues to manage patient care, hospitals would be without qualified personnel to deliver care and public health departments (PHD) would lack professional support to monitor infections, teach prevention and promote health. Nursing has been at the core of the healthcare delivery system just as it has been instrumental in the step-by-step development of colleague disciplines.

Nursing moved forward in the 20th century during the growth of the healthcare industry by becoming organised, educated in institutions of higher education, and extending and advancing nursing practice and health services to all sections of the community. Nursing today, in the US, is well established in the higher education sector, particularly at higher degree level, and advanced level practice continues to develop as demand for healthcare rises. Registration is more problematic, with some qualifications not recognised across state boundaries. This situation is changing, however, largely as a result of pressure from the nurse practitioner movement. In 1995 certification by national professional organisations became a requirement in order to practice in many states.

The development of a particular role of nursing – the nurse practitioner – is explored in detail in Chapter Five. Although many countries now have nurse practitioners in post, it is to the US that we can look for the origins and development of this role. It is believed that by a detailed assessment of the evolution of this advanced nursing role we can more fully understand and more appropriately respond to challenge and change in the future.

Changing practice, through changing the way education is delivered, is the subject of Chapter Six, in which Connors *et al.* provide a rationale for locating nursing education in the community to better meet both the community's health needs and the educational needs of nurses and other health workers as they prepare to practice in this new century.

References

Anderson R, Rice T and Kominski G (1996) *Changing The U.S. Health Care System.* Jossey Bass, San Francisco.

Johnson H and Broder D (1996) *The System: The American Way of Politics at the Breaking Point.* Little Brown, Boston.

Starr P (1982) *The Social Transformation of American Medicine.* Basic Books, New York.

CHAPTER FIVE

The nurse practitioner in the US

Rosemary Goodyear

> *Advanced practice nurses, especially nurse practitioners and certified nurse-midwives, repeatedly have demonstrated their ability to provide cost effective, high quality primary care for many of the neediest members of society.* (Safriet, 1992)

The transitions that have occurred in medicine have given shape to the existing system of delivering healthcare in the US (Starr, 1982). However, scientific discoveries are only one factor in the design of the current US healthcare delivery system. It is the intent of this chapter to explore the historical trends and issues influencing healthcare, describe the development of the nurse practitioner as a provider of healthcare services, and provide several case studies that depict the impact of managed care on this role as it exists today. The rationale for exploring the development of this advanced practice role in detail is that without a view of the past the future cannot be understood.

The development of nursing in the US

The development of nursing at the dawn of the 20th century was marked by the beginning of registration through licensure on a state-by-state basis (New York State was first, in 1900). Laws for registration were usually established after developing a graduate nurses association (Kalisch and Kalisch, 1986). Other states followed, but New York was the more progressive as their law stipulated the education and training requirements that were needed prior to a licence being granted. Postgraduate education in nursing was centred in Teachers College in New York, headed by Adelaide Nutting, who was later to become the leader in preparing nurse educators.

All of these advances took place in an era of reform. Reform of medical and nursing education were only two of the points of change. Growth of the commerce of the country, improved transport and greater personal prosperity brought about this period of social reform. Occupational advancements brought about changes in labour laws that also influenced the working conditions for the nurse. World War I was also a period of advancement for nursing. Educational institutions were called upon to educate nurses to meet the increased demand and this request opened college doors. The different forms of education and work changed the perception of the nurse in the US during and following the war years (Kalisch and Kalisch, 1995). The period after World War I, however, marked an image problem for nurses. The Goldmark Report stressed the need for university education to train nurse leaders, and also addressed the conflict of apprenticeship versus classroom preparation. Educators heeded the discussion and pressed for evaluation and change.

The start of World War II changed the education of nursing by further increasing demand for both the numbers of nurses and expansion of their skills base. The introduction of antibiotics, advances in surgical procedures and an economic boom also influenced the growth of the healthcare industry. The emergence of the Health Maintenance Organisation (HMO), as a form of health insurance, also occurred at this time.

Nursing moved wholeheartedly into collegiate-based education and the rise of the profession flourished. Hospitals were the major employer of nurses and externally controlled the supply and demand for graduates. In the late 1950s and early 1960s the women's movement created an opportunity for multiple groups to come together and support issues of under-representation and recognition of professional issues. Many nurses joined these groups and voiced their protest of under-representation and oppression, some of which could be found in the healthcare industry. Also early in the 1960s the cyclical nursing shortage re-occurred and the government was called upon to resolve the problem (Friss, 1994). A consultant group called by the Surgeon General identified the need for federal support for schools preparing nurses. The expansion of the funds allocated for nurse education through the Nurse Training Act of 1964 was passed by Congress and enacted. The renewal and amended Nurse Training Act occurred in succeeding years 1966, 1968, 1971 and 1975. In addition, the age of advanced technology in healthcare was dawning. Diagnostic and therapeutic advances, harnessing of infectious diseases, along with an increase of heart disease, cancer and stroke placed new demands on nurse education.

Politically the US was experiencing turmoil as a result of the assassination of President Kennedy, the Vietnam War and the passage of two pieces of legislation, Medicare and Medicaid. These new healthcare laws were drafted as an assistance bill for the impoverished and an eligibility bill for the aged. This legislation, passed in 1965, was the second major policy change in the 20th century to shape the healthcare industry. The Social Security Act in 1935 was the first.

New roles for nurses

The role of the nurse was changing as new needs emerged. The clinical nurse specialist, prepared to work in hospitals, was traditionally educated at Master's level. This was also the time (1960s) that the role of the nurse practitioner began. In the University of Colorado doctors Lee Ford and Henry Silver brought together two concepts for preparing nurses who had gained experience in the community. These nurses were to return to study and be introduced to new knowledge and skills that would enable them to meet the increasing demands of patients for health maintenance and health promotion (Ford, 1975):

> My interest was in developing a clinical focus at the advanced level for the family and community nursing curriculum.

This programme prepared the nurse in areas which traditionally had been the domain of the physician. The technical skills of performing a physical exam and the knowledge of eliciting a history, making diagnoses and developing plans of care were not altogether new to nursing, but performing these tasks within the context of the nursing role was new (Ford, 1975):

> We believed the nurse could be a responsible decision maker from a scientific database, collecting data through the use of tools and techniques that had previously been considered the physicians'.

The tools of the stethoscope and sphygmomanometer were developed in 1816 and 1883 respectively, but were not deemed able to be used by nurses until the 1930s, when the skill of taking a blood pressure became part of the nurses' role. So too, the new tools of the ophthalmoscope and otoscope were being handed over to the nurse to perform a more complete assessment and assist the patient achieve a higher level of health. This transition to (previously) 'medical' care was met with scepticism, outrage and doubt by both nursing and medicine. In review of the history of these disciplines we have seen this scenario repeated with regularity as scientific advances and periods of crisis have occurred. Therefore, this response could have been expected; in time the role would become better accepted and progress of the profession would continue. Having a knowledge of history does not, however, make the process any less painful for those experiencing the transition.

The resistance to the role of nurse practitioner can be traced through the literature of both professions (Ford, 1975):

> *In the beginning, we had a great deal of difficulty. There was a problem of territoriality and challenges about who was going to be in charge of pediatric nursing, and all sorts of nonsense.*

The once-solid medical community was experiencing a shift due to diversified funding and interests in healthcare. The academic centres, GPs and public sector physicians were beginning to pursue three different avenues of medicine; research, service and care of the undeserved. The medical community also had divided attention as new policies were being set down in Washington concerning healthcare coverage for the aged and poor as well as broad policies addressing community needs (Starr, 1982). These evolving changes focused the efforts of the medical community on shaping policies that would dictate their fiscal future and not on the development and education of related clinicians.

Education of nurse practitioners

Meanwhile the preparation of nurse practitioners remained controversial, and programmes were based in continuing education (CE) departments within schools of nursing or medicine. Nurse practitioner education was not the only issue confronting nurse educators during this period. Members of the American Nurses Association (ANA) presented a position paper, submitted by their Committee on Education and adopted by the Board of Directors of ANA, which set in motion an ever-widening split among junior college and hospital-based programmes and collegiate-prepared nurses. The position paper (Kalisch and Kalisch, 1986) in essence indicated that the education of:

> *all of those who are licensed to practice nursing should take place in institutions of higher education; minimum preparation for beginning professional nursing practice should be a baccalaureate degree; minimum preparation for beginning technical nursing practice should be an associate degree in nursing; education for assistants in the health service occupations should be short intensive pre service programs in vocational education rather than on-the-job training.*

In the minds of many this created a professional elitism; only individuals prepared in institutions of higher education were practising professionally. A broader implication for schools of nursing was the potential demise of hospital programmes, preparing diploma nurses. This was perceived as a denial of nursing's roots. Thus, the emergence of a clinician who embraced knowledge and skills previously ascribed to medicine still posed a different threat to the profession.

Nursing within the larger arena of reform was supportive of services for the minority and ageing populations. Since nursing traditionally had been linked with serving the underserved they were very vocal in many of the issues being debated in Washington. This stance placed nursing and medicine on opposite sides in the public policy forum, with medicine maintaining the status quo of private practice and fee for service without governmental intervention, and nursing speaking out for reform that would provide governmental support for healthcare of the aged and poor.

The preparation of the nurse practitioner continued to emerge in two centres in the US: the University of Colorado with doctors Ford and Silver, and the University of Rochester in New York where Kitzman and Hoekelman were also looking at the expansion of the nurse's role in the paediatric setting. Bates, a physician on the faculty at the University of Rochester wrote (1972):

> . . . *our healthcare system is seriously outmoded and nursing holds the answer . . . each health profession carves its own role, identifying those needs to which it will address its knowledge, skill and efforts . . . The role of each is in part unique, and in part overlapping with others.*

More recently another non-nurse repeated this concept when in 1992 Barbara Safriet dedicated an issue of the *Yale Journal on Regulation* to addressing the under-utilisation of nurse practitioners as a means of resolving the spiralling cost of healthcare. She further discussed the restraint in achieving their full potential, due in part to the regulating agencies across the nation (Safriet, 1992):

> *Advanced practice nurses, especially nurse practitioners and certified nurse-midwives, repeatedly have demonstrated their ability to provide cost effective, high quality primary care for many of the neediest members of society.*

In the early 1970s a proliferation of programmes preparing nurse practitioners at the CE level were started. The appearance of programmes educating nurse practitioners at the Master's level did not evolve until later in the decade. Questions arising out of a 'professional' as opposed to a 'technical' nurse, and the nurse practitioner as a clinician, generated a volume of research into roles, curricula, quality of care and theory development which has not been matched since. It was an era that also saw nurse leaders espousing positions related to these issues, which also has not been repeated. Many camps were established and this made for an extremely tumultuous era in nursing. The nurse practitioner is one of the lasting symbols of this time of change. The educational issues of professional versus technical nursing remain unresolved, but have been tailored by economic support and public policy (Friss, 1994).

Curricula

Curricular guidelines were essentially non-existent in the early years of nurse practitioner education. The coalescing of supportive physicians and nurses to develop a programme on sound educational principles was a first step in the evolution of nurse practitioner education. The obvious areas of content were easily identified, such as health history and physical examination. The merging of content to teach nurses about the management of patient illnesses was more difficult. Many nursing programmes began with supportive physician colleagues determining the course content that nurse practitioners would need to provide service in an ambulatory care setting. Common health problems presenting in the ambulatory settings, differences between socio-economic levels, as well as racial and ethnic populations were discussed and considered. Since many diverse populations settled in the US, these factors had to be incorporated in the curricula. The inclusion of content crucial for nurses to operate efficiently and effectively as critical thinkers and decision makers was also essential. Technology in teaching and simulated situations facilitated the process of providing students with sample patients so that they could develop a level of competence prior to working within the actual clinical settings.

The first curricula consisted of courses on health history, physical examination, management of common health problems, pharmaco-therapeutics, nursing issues, role and clinical practice. The family nurse practitioner programmes included sessions on family theory, clinical experience in monitoring families in the community, case management of patients over long-term and experience of encountering and caring for individuals across the lifespan. The implementation of this content was dependent on the educational site of the nurse practitioner programmee. Programmes based in the departments of continuing education tended to be condensed and intense in the amount of content provided in a short period of time. Programmes taught at the Master's level in universities had a longer timeframe and stressed the theoretical foundation, research and core courses prior to moving into the management and clinical components. The guidelines for developing programmes were first issued by ANA and consisted of eight pages (ANA, 1975). Today guidelines for nurse practitioner pro-grammes have been developed by an organisation specifically devoted to the education of the nurse practitioner known as the National Organ-ization of Nurse Practitioner Faculties (NONPF). These guidelines cover many pages and are much more detailed (NONPF, 1995).

A controversy between nurse educators preparing nurse practitioners and educators of traditional nurses was the perception that the expanded scope of practice was not nursing. The new curriculum content was viewed as medicine and therefore did not belong in schools of higher education or in the curricula of traditional nursing. These nurse leaders chose to disregard the successful actions of nurses in combat during the wars as well as the added skills and technique nurses were performing within hospitals. These procedures were part of advanced technology and were seen as an exception to the role and performed under the direction of a physician. The nurse practitioner, however, was viewed as outside these boundaries (Rogers, 1983) and:

> *nurses who . . . become physician's assistants or pediatric associates must realize that they are leaving nursing.*

Another factor, although not documented in the nursing literature, was the large amount of funding received from the federal government under the Nurse Training Act. These funds were provided to educate nurse practitioners at the certificate level in continuing education programmes. The inclusion of the educational programmes into tradi-tional graduate education would therefore reduce the revenues that were available to schools and colleges of nursing. All administrators know that any programme with a strong clinical component is extremely expensive to operate (Friss, 1994). In addition, and in defence of academia, there were insufficient numbers of qualified faculty to teach nurse practitioners and physician support was needed. Eventually funds were available through the Nurse Training Act to prepare faculty as nurse practitioners and this assisted in the transition of nurse practitioner programmes moving into the Master's level. Research into the placement of these programmes was conducted prior to these changes (Hoekelman *et al.*, 1975; Linn, 1976; Sultz *et al.*, 1976; Jelinek, 1978).

Political organisation and autonomy

At a conference on primary care held in Kansas City in 1974 entitled 'Building for the Future', a group of nurse practitioners joined together and listed issues and concerns they wanted the ANA to address in their upcoming meetings. The issues identified were: enlisting the National Joint Practice Committee to respond to the needs of the nurse practitioner; liaison and communication with other existing practice councils; establishing a clearing house for information for nurse practitioners; and beginning discussion on the feasibility of a national exam for nurse practitioners (Kelley and Clancy, 1974, personal communication). Meanwhile nurse practitioners were testifying at legislative committee hearings convened for the purpose of studying reimbursement and their expanded role. These committees were investigating the most economical method for providing needed health services to the low income and impoverished residents of medically underserved areas of the US. In one programme the nurses prepared as family nurse practitioners reported that 98% of the graduates returned and remained working in rural underserved communities in Texas (Goodyear, 1978). The same statement could not be supported by the medical school graduates, as they did not return to the rural areas following completion of their schooling.

In 1971, in the report commissioned by the Secretary of Health, Education and Welfare, a group studied extending the scope of nursing practice (Richardson, 1971) and related that they believed:

> . . . the future of nursing must encompass a substantially larger place within the community of the health professions. Moreover, we believe that extending the scope of nursing practice is essential if this nation is to achieve the goal of equal access to health services for all its citizens . . .

The commission's report addressed educational, legal and inter-professional relationships between physicians and nurses as well as the impact on healthcare delivery. In essence they encouraged curric-ular innovations to demonstrate the concept of a physician–nurse team in the delivery of healthcare, the orderly transfer of responsibilities between medicine and nursing, and collaboration between schools of medicine and nursing to demonstrate effective interaction. It also directed the implementation of cost-benefit analyses and similar stud-ies in settings where nurses were delivering care in the extended role. This landmark report can be identified, in the political arena, as the issue that promoted the Rural Health Clinics Act 95-210 which was passed by Congress in 1977, and was signed into law as the first act to mandate reimbursement for nurse practitioner services. This law allowed the clinics in the rural communities to bill the state and federal governments and receive reimbursement for nurse practitioner services without requiring a physician signature or billing authorisa-tion. This was also viewed as another step in the autonomy of the nurse practitioner as a provider of healthcare, and the advancement of nursing in the US.

Standards of practice and credentialling

In the 1970s, about ten years after the introduction of nurse practitioner education, the educators and practitioners identified a need to establish consistency in preparation as well as outcomes. An examination to measure the competency of graduates was proposed. A group of concerned nurse practitioner educators raised the plausibility of such a test with representatives of ANA and asked them to explore the options and methods for initiating such a test. The variety of pro-grammes, different programme lengths and no consistent curriculum threatened the credibility of the nurse practitioner. Thus the first certification examinations by a professional organisation, external to institutions of higher education and state licensing boards, was insti-tuted. ANA, the professional organisation representing the practice issues of all nurses in the US, had taken a role in guiding the development of this group of clinicians, since they were essentially homeless and unclaimed in terms of an educational base. At this time the Council of State Boards of Nursing had not issued any statement regarding the competency of nurse practitioners. They were assessing the breadth of the Nurse Practice Acts, the legal basis for a licenced clinician to practice and determining if nurse practitioners could practice within the boundaries of their respective state. Twenty years later, in 1995, certification by national professional organisations became a requirement in order to practice in many states across the nation. This transition from establishing credibility as a new clinician seeking a measure of competence to setting a standard of practice demonstrates another lasting symbol of professional change brought about by the nurse practitioner movement.

The credentialling examinations, first started by ANA in 1975, have been changed from a day and a half of testing, to half a day of testing in 1997. Today the focus is on clinical management with testing carried out on computer. This change has been brought about by the need for the certificate examination to be able to withstand legal scrutiny in the courts, and competing certification examinations by specialty groups. The requirement of all nurse practitioners to be prepared at the Master's level, in an accredited programme, has helped make the knowledge uniform and testable. Development of curricular guidelines by the NONPF has been instrumental in guiding programmes to prepare nurse practitioners at a level of competence in graduate education. They have worked with accrediting bodies, faculties and governmental agencies with the aim of achieving this goal.

Credentialling in the US is complex. The country is made up of 50 states, therefore 50 different Boards of Nursing. In most instances a nurse must be licensed and registered before s/he can pursue an education as a nurse practitioner. The nurse must also possess a Bachelor's degree in nursing or an allied health field in order to be admitted into the graduate programmes of most major universities. In addition s/he must adhere to the scope of practice in the state of residence as stipulated by the Board of Nursing. Upon graduation from the Masters programme, the State Board of Nursing can also require additional criteria for practising as a nurse practitioner, or as more currently referred to, an Advanced Practice Nurse (APN). The function of the State Board of Nursing is to protect the public and assure that anyone describing themselves as a nurse practitioner is safe and competent to practice.

The evolution of a new role historically begins with a demand for new knowledge and skill from the practice arena, then educational institutions create new programmes to meet these needs; the final phase of legitimisation is the legal arm that protects the public, by establishing criteria for the newly defined professional or scope of practice. The trend in the US today is to recognise the needs of the mobile professional society, and to pilot a multi-state licensure so that nurses can practise using a license recognised in more than one state.

Managed care and the rise of nurse practitioners

Managed care was initiated in response to the consumer's dissatisfaction with the healthcare system in the 1990s. The public sent the message that government intervention was no longer desirable as a method to correct the problem. The selection for private industry to have an opportunity to improve the system was supported. This shift in thinking and policy brought about a search by the insurance industry, and big business, for cost-reducing mechanisms that had not previously been used. Personnel, being the biggest expense next to new technology, were a target for review and analysis. The managed care companies researched the successful staff model, HMOs, and identified that the nurse practitioner had a history of providing quality, cost-effective care.

Suddenly this clinician was in tremendous demand. Positions in these managed care companies abounded. Salaries which had been stagnant soared, and schools of nursing were pressured by this industry to generate more graduates. Schools of nursing across the US who previously had not undertaken preparation of this clinician suddenly started programmes. The federal funds which had been allocated for preparation of nurse practitioners were being over-solicited, schools opened programmes without sufficient qualified faculty and in one state nurses graduated from institutions that had not been approved to prepare them. This cycle of nursing shortage at one end of the continuum was triggered by the downsizing of hospitals and the release of nurses due to fewer hospital admissions. For the first time in decades the graduate nurse had to be innovative in securing a position or return to school. The influx of Master's-prepared nurses into nurse practitioner programmes lasted for approximately three years. The job market in many states is now flooded with nurse practitioners and competition for positions is now driving the once lucrative salaries back down to what they were prior to the shortage.

The physician and the nurse practitioner in many states were competing for the same position. However, state regulation and reimbursement limited the nurse practitioner's scope of practice. Reimbursement for nurse practitioner services can only be accessed through their employer, an MCO, a physician, a group of physicians or a hospital. The nurse practitioner cannot be a primary care provider (PCP) under managed care even though this is in conflict with many state laws (Academy Update, 1999). Nurse practitioners had, in the past, received payment for their services through federally funded

programmes such as Medicaid and federal employee insurance programmes, but the MCOs, a corporate entity, do not have to abide by
these rules. This issue is currently unresolved and nurse practitioners
are being excluded from direct reimbursement by the MCOs. Policies
addressing this exclusion are being promulgated, but there is less
chance they will be quickly changed in states where a strong medical
association is in place.

Delivering change: three nursing case studies

Nurse practitioners deliver a good, safe service, are good value for
money and are respected and used by the public. The history of their
employment substantiates this.

Health Science Centers (HSCs) have been a major employer of nurse
practitioners since the introduction of the role in the 1960s. HSCs are
the setting where health professionals are educated, technologies are
introduced and services for the uninsured are provided. Historically
these institutions had a rotating medical student population and the
nurse practitioner was initially intended to provide services for minor
health problems and allow the medical student to focus on major,
complex problems. Soon after this role was accepted in the HSC
hospitals and clinics they discovered that the nurse practitioner was
the most stable personnel, the best received and the most plausible to
manage the complex and long-term patients. This finding was true in
the internal medical, family practice, and paediatric clinics within the
HSCs. It was also true in the HMOs, group practices and community
clinics. Thus the nurse practitioner became the consistent primary care
provider who afforded continuity for the patients and security for the
individual with long-term health problems.

Other strengths emerged as the nurse practitioner demonstrated an
ability to communicate at the level of the patient, educate the patient
about their illness and consider the whole patient, presenting their
problem and not just the disease. A fuller picture of this area of work is
provided by presentation of three case studies drawn from practice and
shown below.

Nurse One

Nurse One is a nurse practitioner prepared initially in a certificate programme, then pursuing a Master of Nursing degree. Her professional nursing history includes being a public health nurse in a culturally diverse, low economic community setting. Nurse Practitioner One's (NP1) return to education was stimulated by the demand for more and more complex decisions regarding the health problems presenting in the clinics. In addition, demands by the agency to manage these patients, as there were no other resources available for patient care, encouraged educational pursuits. As one of the first students in a new certificate programme preparing nurse practitioners in the mid-1970s her education was based in a HSC and concentrated in a three-month period for classroom and clinical content. Following this time an approved preceptorship with a physician preceptor was established and continued for the next nine months in her community of origin. NP1 was on the frontier of change in the state and under much scrutiny for taking on this new role. She had to explain constantly (as did her classmates) what a nurse practitioner did and why they did not just go to medical school. Strong preceptor support was identified as being of major assistance during the period of role development in this community and in this state. The recognition that a graduate degree was needed to grow professionally and assure credibility for the services that were being provided accompanied the nurse practitioner's pursuit of a Master's degree.

From her original position in a health department, NP1 transferred to a major HSC in Minnesota, the Mayo Clinic. There, in the department of paediatrics this clinician established the role of the nurse practitioner provider, sought out by the physicians and their families as their primary care provider. Clinical services and mentoring medical students in the art of providing primary care became one of her strengths. After 14 years of positive clinical practice she moved to another HSC on the west coast and, in collaboration with a physician, established a role in the care of children with multiple health problems. These children had neurological, developmental and environmental insults that manifest themselves as delayed development, as well as other complex problems. The role of mentor and teacher of medical students rotating through this specialty was also incorporated into NP1's position at this HSC. The participation in decisions to operate the programme, provide and participate in educational conferences while maintaining a focus on quality care were strengths and benefits of this position.

After almost 20 years of practice as a nurse practitioner the changes introduced by managed care had altered the direction of this clinician's career. The HSCs were forced to downsize staff in the wake of fiscal exigencies. They offered long-time personnel the option to contract externally for part of their salary. NP1 accepted the option and contracted for one year with a large physician group practice that focused on children with allergic disorders. This change encompassed a move from a large, non-profitable public institution to a profit-making private group practice. Security and longevity were issues that had to be considered and this one-year contract allowed NP1 to test out the new setting while the group of physicians experienced the nurse practitioner providing services in their setting. These physicians had known NP1 and had attempted to hire her away from the HSC for three years, but the downsizing forced the issue and a new job had to be considered. Concerns that the nurse clinician had prior to making this transition were as follows.

- Would patients accept the clinician in a private practice setting?
- What tasks and positions would the clinician fill since the practice was made up of only physicians?
- How would decisions be made about the operations of the practice?
- How is professional growth and development managed in this setting?

The acceptance of NP1 into the practice was accomplished by the physicians introducing the clinician as a new member of the group and explaining that she would be also be 'seeing' patients. Many of the patients knew about nurse practitioners and they had no qualms about being managed by NP1. This was a very different experience for NP1 than she had as a new nurse practitioner 20 years earlier. Then the patients came from poor populations with limited resources, whereas in this position she would be providing services to affluent, highly insured populations.

There were some losses as a result of leaving the HSC; inclusion as a researcher, the collegiality of fellow NPs, involvement in programme development, continuing education and being able to provide health-care regardless of concern about the cost or patient income were all cited as not present in the new setting. However, the career interruption of managed (for profit) care, together with peer physician support, has opened other opportunities for this clinician. She is expanding the role to include operating an office in the absence of the physicians, opening another office in another part of the community, and speaking to local and national groups about managing paediatric patients with respiratory and allergic conditions. This nurse practitioner was, potentially, a casualty of the managed care transition, but was successful in moving from the public to the private sector (without loss of status or income) because she possessed 20 years' successful experience as a nurse practitioner, and the knowledge and skills to predict and manage change.

Nurse Two

Nurse Two, a public health nurse (PHN) for more than 20 years, has often experienced change and most recently as a result of the introduction of managed care. In the US the PHN is often viewed as providing services for low-income and impoverished populations. These patients are frequently enrolled in the federal and state programmes of Medicaid and/or Medicare. The services, however, are available to and cover all residents with a focus on health maintenance, health promotion, disease prevention and environmental services. Traditionally the surveillance of communicable disease and monitoring health hazards has always been provided by the Public Health Departments (PHD). However, over the last two decades, federal and state programmes aimed at assuring access to healthcare have been allowed to expand and include primary care services. In communities where sufficient numbers of willing physician providers were not available, the federal government ascribed the designation of 'medically underserved' and/or 'medical shortage area'. It was in these communities that the PHD first initiated primary care clinics in conjunction with the traditional services.

The PHNs were some of the first applicants in nurse practitioner programms in the late 1960s and early 1970s. This trend was in line with the thinking of Dr Ford, who envisioned the PHN to be in a perfect position to fulfil this new role. Health departments (HDs), especially in rural communities and cities with large numbers of impoverished people, were eager to have the PHN prepared with these new skills and assessment abilities. HD programmes were funded to include gathering data of health histories, screening physicals, anticipatory guidance, patient education and referral. Two programmes that demonstrate the fulfilment of the mission of public health while incorporating the nurse prepared as a nurse practitioner are known as EPSDT and WIC. The Early Periodic Screening and Developmental Testing programme focused on assessing children between newborn and 21 years of age, providing anticipatory guidance for the parents, immunisations and testing. The Women, Infant and Children programme included assessing pregnant women and providing education on nutrition during and following pregnancy. Vouchers for nutritious food were also provided following educational sessions, and special formulas needed by infants unable to tolerate the regular formula feedings. In some communities these programmes broke the ground for the initiation of primary care services in the health departments. The populations being served were largely uninsured or working poor without health insurance benefits, thus unattractive to the primary care physician.

These screening programmes started in the 1970s and continue today. In some areas the health departments are contracting with MCOs to continue these services since the primary care physician will not accept these patients. When the physician accepts these publically insured patients they often sub-contract for these screening services, since they are very time consuming and the reimbursement does not cover the cost of their time. However, the premise that the primary care physician is the professional to treat illnesses still persists today. The closing of primary care services in the health departments has largely been due to a reallocation of funding with the onset of MCOs.

MCOs ushered in the reordering of government funding. The governmental policy makers at the national level were directed to develop plans for distributing funds to the states and not to the specific programmes or communities. Thus the redistribution has brought about different priorities in each state's spending regarding the public health needs of their citizens. In many states this coincided with placing all primary care services within the managed care framework to be distributed to primary care providers. These were privately funded programmes as well as publicly funded programmes. The result was that health departments were excluded from entering into these contracts and funding for primary care services was no longer available. This system makes it inevitable that inequalities in healthcare will occur.

Managed care has redirected not only the funding of programmes, but the role of the PHN as well. The second scenario focuses on the role of a PHN who has served in the PHDs as a clinician caring in part for a special population with Hansen's disease. Since the largest number of clients served by this PHN (a graduate with a Master's degree in nursing) are from the Medicare and Medicaid programmes, her major responsibility has been to oversee the transition of these patients into managed care programmes. Refocusing of the services of the health department, advocating for patients who do not understand the changes, and supporting staff in this time of transition make up the current role of the PHN. Programmes of home visiting, case management and direct primary care service have given way to surveillance, monitoring and assurance of a healthy population. The role of this PHN, as an administrator, is to guide other PHNs in their new duties of acting as a mediator, referral resource and translator of information about the choice and process of managed care plan. They have had to spend a great deal of preparation time to become experts in this transition process, not necessarily what their education has prepared them to do. In some instances a major role is to be sure the patient does not fall through the cracks of the changing system, but gains access to the appropriate provider to have their health needs met. An example of nursing intervention is assuring that children receive the appropriate vaccines when a contracted provider does not have adequate storage facilities available. The PHN will spend time educating the staff of the private provider, or referring the parent and child to an appropriate facility. In such instances the MCO must sub-contract with an appropriate provider.

It is worth commenting here that although this is a time of disruption, it can also be seen as a time of opportunity. Innovative PHNs will be able to identify needs that are unmet with the transition and initiate policy to allow the services of the health departments to continue. This challenge comes at the beginning of the 21st century just as a similar challenge to facilitate care for the influx of immigrants came at the beginning of the 20th century in the tenements of New York City.

Nurse Three

The nurse practitioner in private practice provides yet another scenario of the role during changes in the healthcare system in the US. A rural community serving a population of farmers and farmworkers provided an opportunity for a family nurse practitioner (FNP) to start a private practice. The local hospital and medical community had failed at initiating an outreach site in a growing community ten miles from the hospital. The FNP researched the opportunity, legal parameters, invested in a community survey and explored the plausibility of initiating a practice with the medical community. Colleague nurse practitioners were supportive in the discussion and planning phases of establishing the practice. The intent was to initiate a practice site where nurse practitioners could explore opportunities for beginning a practice of their own once sufficient clients had been amassed.

Starting a private practice without a model or mentor is stressful and risky. The research and knowledge of business that clinicians must accrue on their own can be overwhelming and time consuming. The need for experts in areas of business and law was identified early in the process and they were contracted so that all necessary negotiations could be assessed and appropriately managed. The hospital facilitated the establishment of the practice by sub-leasing space for the practice.

A medical director was contracted so that the full scope of practice as a nurse practitioner could be implemented under the existing rules and regulations of the state. In addition three additional consultants in paediatrics, family practice, and obstetrics and gynaecology were contracted as back-up support for the practice.

Public information and advertisement were other areas foreign to the nurse practitioner. Experts in these fields were also hired to let the community know this new health service would soon be available. Perhaps the most difficult part of this undertaking was to come to terms with the type of service that would be available. Putting one's philosophy of care into business terms that the consumer can understand, grasp and enrol in is difficult. The next difficult task is implementing this level of practice in an entirely new and competitive environment. Education in traditional nursing programmes does not encompass these concepts or processes.

Many weeks of hard work followed to secure equipment, supplies and personnel. Funds were quickly depleted and minimal income marked the first year of practice. The fact that nurse practitioners could be reimbursed only under the auspices of the medical director became very clear. The practice was owned and operated by an FNP, but reimbusement for services could only be collected through the signature or identification code of the MD. Private and public insurances followed the same guidelines and only two federally supported health programmes reimbursed nurse practitioners directly. In rural communities the number of fee-for-service patients were insufficient to support the practice. The decision to contract for Medicaid patients specifically for EPSDT patients was supported by the medical director since none of the medical community accepted these publically insured patients in their private practices. This decision became the opportunity for the FNP to demonstrate fiscal autonomy in the years to come.

Patients seeking services gradually learned of the practice and their numbers continued to grow. Women and children made up the largest group of patients in this practice. Collaboration with the local school, migrant workers and public health nurses helped to build and gain recognition within the community. Federal laws were amended to allow direct reimbursement to nurse practitioners for patients enrolled in Medicaid programmes in all states. The regulation had to be changed, however, in each state before the law came into effect. This process took four years.

Several nurse practitioner colleagues worked with the FNP to build the practice, and nurse practitioner students from a university programme were mentored in the practice. The role of the nurse practitioner in interdependent practice was being modelled. A unique entrepreneur experience was available for student learning while skills and critical thinking exercises were being tested with each patient. It was a laboratory where a few students were able to gain insight into the role and domain of a nurse practitioner in private practice.

The relationship the FNP establishes with patients selecting the practice as their primary care site is difficult to describe: following family members during a pregnancy to school entrance, a mother through a miscarriage and then through a successful delivery, or a woman through a distressed perimenopausal period to hormonal balance can be expressed in words but words fall short in relating the actual experience. The trust between the nurse practitioner and the patient is weighted with responsibility, accountability, respect and competence on the part of the clinician and responsibility, dependability and honesty on the part of the patient and family. These build with each encounter and become the foundation for the patient–clinician relationship. This trust overcomes language, age, racial and cultural differences and allows a level of communication to take place that is easily understood by all parties.

A potential threat to practice, the change in the healthcare system, was observed early and plans to link up with a larger organisation were attempted from 1992 to 1995. Organisations were disinterested about merging with a private practice that focused on health maintenance. Additionally, policy makers were not concerned with the individual clinician, but focused their work on enrolling all residents of the state in some form of managed healthcare plan. The nurse practitioner was politically aware of the events, but no system wanted to deal with a practice that only served the publically insured patients. Policy did change in 1993 however, and direct billing for services rendered by a nurse practitioner to Medicaid patients was activated. The efforts of nurse legislators, colleagues in the professional organisations and continual requests to the policy makers facilitated this change in the regulations – another success for the nurse practitioner in one state.

There were further difficulties ahead, however. The transition of enrolling Medicaid patients into managed care began to draw off many of the patients from the practice. The assignments into MCOs by the welfare system became a standard event and the patients, many of whom were non-English speaking, did not know how to make their selection known. The fact that a nurse practitioner could not be identified as a PCP had become a reality and the next barrier in private practice. The policy makers were listening to the clinicians of power. These clinicians were the physicians and only certain physicians were able to be identified as PCPs.

At the turn of the 21st century, nine years after the practice was started, this issue remains unresolved. The practice was closed after six years of active successful service to a community of over 500 families. These families have had to be placed with other practices in the community or in the surrounding community. The economists would not consider this endeavour a success, and the physicians would indicate the same. However, the nurse practitioner, colleagues, students and patients see positive outcomes. The demonstration was of a nurse practitioner, initiating and implementing a private practice based on a nursing model, providing unparalleled service for a period of six years.

Managed care has altered the delivery of healthcare in the US, establishing new and different criteria for the clinicians and changing the method of reimbursement for service. These changes have resulted in shutting out nurse practitioners as primary care providers, for the time being. Their experience, however has fuelled the desire to share their story and to motivate future nurse entrepreneurs in the 21st century.

Conclusions

The development of the nurse practitioner role has made a significant contribution to healthcare in the US. There are lessons here that might be instructive for other countries as they seek to develop this advanced practice nursing role. Particular attention should be paid to the way in which professional organisation, appropriate education, setting of standards and credentialling have been achieved.

Although lacking formal education in business and entrepreneurial skills, US nurses demonstrate a high level of political awareness and flexibility; in many instances this has paid off; in some instances they remain limited by external factors such as the expansion of the healthcare market, protectionist professional practices and restrictive legislation.

Market forces are driving healthcare in the US. There are opportunities for nurses, in alliances with others, to benefit. Consumers are demanding an improved and less costly healthcare system. Nurse practitioners have shown that they are good value for money, deliver effective services, are liked by the public, and reach out to all sectors of society. Working in large medical centres, public health agencies and private practice they daily demonstrate the success of their role. They should be supported in their endeavours.

References

Academy Update (1999) *Managed Care Legislation*. American Academy of Nurse Practitioners, Austin, TX.

American Nurses Association (1975) *Guidelines for short-term continuing education programs preparing adult and family nurse practitioners*. ANA Council of Family Nurse Practitioners and Clinicians. CH-4 3M: 1–8.

Bates B (1972) *Nurse Physician Dyad: Collegial or Competitive?* Selected Papers from the 1972 ANA Convention, 30 April–5 May, Detroit.

Ford L (1975) An interview with Dr Loretta Ford. *The Nurse Practitioner: A Journal of Primary Care Nursing* **1**(1): 9.

Friss L (1994) Nursing studies laid end to end form a circle. *Journal of Health Politics, Policy and Law* **19**(3): 597–631.

Goodyear R (1978) Special Subcommittee on Rural Health Care Services: Nurse Practitioners – Health Care Providers in Texas. Lieutenant Governor's Committee Room, State Capitol, Austin, TX.

Hoekelman RN *et al.* (1975) *An evaluation of preparation of pediatric nurse practitioners*. Unpublished monograph, University of Rochester, Rochester, NY.

Jelinek D (1978) The longitudinal study of nurse practitioners: report of phase II. *Nurse Practitioner Journal* **3**(1): 17–19.

Kalisch P and Kalisch B (1986) *The Advance of American Nursing* (2e). Little Brown, Boston.

Kalisch P and Kalisch B (1995) *The Advance of American Nursing* (3e). Lippincott, Philadelphia.

Linn L (1976) Type of nursing education and the nurse practitioner experiences. *Nurse Practitioner* **3**(1): 28–33.

NONPF Curriculum Guidelines Task Force (1995) *Curriculum Guidelines & Program Standards for Nurse Practitioner Education: Advanced Nursing Practice*. Washington, DC.

Richardson E (1971) *Extending the Scope of Nursing Practice: A Report of the Secretary's Committee to Study Extended Roles for Nurses*. US Department of Health, Education and Welfare, Washington DC.

Rogers M (1983) Beyond the horizon. In: NL Chaska (ed) *The Nursing Profession: A Time to Speak*. McGraw-Hill, New York.

Safriet B (1992) Health care dollars and regulatory sense: the role of advanced practice nursing. *Yale Journal on Regulation* **9**(2): 417–87.

Starr P (1982) *The Social Transformation of American Medicine*. Basic Books, New York.

Sultz H, Zielenzy M and Kingon L (1976) *Longitudinal Study of Nurse Practitioners, Phase I*. US Government Printing Office, Washington, DC.

CHAPTER SIX

Improving the preparation of nursing professionals through community–campus partnerships

Kara M Connors, Joanne Kirk Henry and Sarena D Seifer

> (it is): *the coming together of these two notions: our innate desire to contribute and our desire to learn as human beings.*
> (Sigmon, quoted in Seifer, 1997)

Introduction

Nursing education in the US is at an exciting place. With dramatic changes taking place in the US healthcare system, today's nursing professionals are increasingly expected to shift from traditional practice in acute care settings and adopt effective practice skills for care in community-based settings. While this path may be less familiar, current political and economic trends in the US leave nursing professionals with few choices. In an effort to shed light on strategies for preparing nursing educators and their students for this new change in practice, the authors will discuss the emerging role of 'service–learning' as an innovative methodology for improving nursing education. The integration of a broader definition of service in academic activity can result in an exciting blend of the traditional teaching–research–service model.

This chapter begins with a rationale justifying the emergence of nursing education in the community. This rationale sets the stage for discussing national strategies for improving student education and community health, and provides an overview of service–learning in health professionals' education. Following an overview of service–learning, the authors examine a nursing service–learning case study, and conclude with a series of recommendations for advancing service–learning in nursing education.

The rationale for the community–campus movement in the United States

Traditionally, the level of educational involvement in community-based settings is reflective of the changing political, economic and social climate of the time. In response to today's rapidly changing healthcare system, the climate of higher education, and the important role faculty plays in developing future student leaders, nursing educators are in a unique position to become more fully engaged in the community. These issues, described in more detail below, contribute to building the rationale for nursing schools' engagement in community-based education.

The healthcare climate in the United States

The American healthcare system is experiencing greater change than any other industry in the country. For more than a decade, the costs of the system have not been bearable; the nation spends over $3000 of its healthcare dollars on individuals when no other nation spends more than $2000 per person (O'Neil, 1998). Despite a trillion dollar investment of healthcare resources, there are 43 million individuals in the US who are uninsured, and one million who join this rank each month (O'Neil, 1998). As healthcare costs continue to rise, the US has witnessed a growing emergence of complex health and social problems. Teen pregnancy, HIV and AIDS, substance use, domestic and gang-related violence, a growing elderly population, and demographic shifts of diverse populations challenge the way healthcare is defined, and where and how it is provided. While healthcare has typically been delivered in expensive, acute-care hospital settings, the effort to contain costs in today's managed care system has meant a dramatic shift towards providing care in co-ordinated and less-expensive community and ambulatory care settings. A key component of containing costs has been the education and training of healthcare professionals to work effectively in teams with other traditional and non-traditional health-care providers. As disorientating as this shift may be to consumers and providers alike, there are underlying forces or 'tensions' that may best explain this movement within the healthcare system. Seifer and O'Neil (cited in Seifer and Connors, 1997) present what they've called 'dynamic tensions in healthcare'. These are illustrated in Table 6.1.

Table 6.1: Dynamic tensions in healthcare

Current paradigm		Emerging paradigm
Specialised care	à	Primary care
Technologically driven	à	Humanely balanced
Cost unaware	à	Cost aware
Institutionally based	à	Community based
Governed professionally	à	Governed managerially
Acute treatment	à	Chronic management
Individual patient focused	à	Population perspective
Curative care	à	Preventive orientation
Individual provider	à	Team provider
Competition	à	Cooperation

Seifer and O'Neil argue that this shift from left to right will heighten the:

> 'attractiveness' of health professions institutions' investment in the health of their surrounding communities through community service and education. In the future, the most valued students entering the health care workforce will be those who are prepared to know more things in broad ways, and to transfer this knowledge in more collaborative teams in community-based settings.

The policy implications for community–campus partnerships

The tensions described by Seifer and O'Neil have created a new set of expectations and demands for future nursing professionals. In response, various health policy leaders and experts have delivered a 'call for action' to health professions schools to develop greater and improved community competencies among their students. The Pew Health Professions Commission, a national blue-ribbon panel of healthcare leaders, believes that health professional schools:

> *must lead the effort to realign training and education to be more consistent with the changing needs of the delivery system.*

This effort can be achieved by adopting the 21 core competencies identified in Box 6.1 by the Commission for the Effective Practice of Nursing and Other Health Professionals.

To realise this vision articulated by the Commission and other policy leaders, the next generation of nurses must be educated in community settings that allow nursing students to provide continuity of care for clients in outpatient settings; practice health promotion and disease prevention strategies; develop client communication and negotiation skills with diverse populations; and deal with social, financial and ethical aspects of care. These community-based experiences will emerge only through meaningful curriculum revision and the development of new partnerships and alliances between nursing schools and community partners, including community health centres, ambulatory clinics, social service agencies, public schools and others.

Shifting expectations and demands on nursing professionals and the schools that have trained them have raised concerns about the strategies for supporting these institutions in adapting to change within the curriculum and community. In response, a growing number of community–campus initiatives and organisations across the country, such as the Health Professions Schools in Service to the Nation Program (HPSISN) and Community–Campus Partnerships for Health (CCPH), have emerged to support health professions schools and communities in managing these changes. Their efforts, discussed in the following section, provide potential solutions for improving student education and the health of communities.

Box 6.1: Effective practice (Pew Health Professions Commission, 1995)

The health professional should:
- embrace a personal ethic of social responsibility and service
- exhibit ethical behaviour in all professional activities
- provide evidence-based, clinically competent care
- incorporate the multiple determinants of health in clinical care
- apply knowledge of the new sciences
- demonstrate critical thinking, reflection and problem-solving skills
- understand the role of primary care
- rigorously practice preventative healthcare
- integrate population-based care and services into practice
- improve access to healthcare for those with unmet health needs
- practice relationship-centred care with individuals and families
- provide culturally sensitive care to a diverse society
- partner with communities in healthcare decisions
- use communication and information technology effectively and appropriately
- work in interdisciplinary teams
- ensure care that balances individual, professional, system and societal needs
- practice leadership
- take responsibility for quality of care and health outcomes at all levels
- contribute to continuous improvement of the healthcare system
- advocate for public policy that promotes and protects the health of the public
- continue to learn and help others learn.

The HPSISN programme and CCPH: strategies to improve student education and community health

The HPSISN programme (1995–1998), a programme of the Pew Health Professions Commission and the National Fund for Medical Education, and supported by The Pew Charitable Trusts, the Corporation for

National Service, and the Health Resources and Services Administration, awarded service–learning grants to 20 health professions schools across the country. The goal of the HPSISN programme was to integrate service–learning into health professions curriculum. The HPSISN grantees included schools of medicine, dentistry, nursing, pharmacy and public health whose community partners represented public schools, community health centres, community development corporations and social service agencies and others. As part of the programme, a national conference was held in 1996 at Northeastern University in Boston, Massachusetts. This conference generated the discussion of a new organisation that would serve as a 'home' for the community–campus partnership movement. This organisation emerged as Community–Campus Partnerships for Health (CCPH) and was officially launched (as a non-profit organisation) in 1997.

The mission of CCPH is to foster partnerships between communities and educational institutions that build on each other's strengths and develop their roles as change agents for improving health professions education, civic responsibility, and the overall health of communities. Based at the Center for the Health Professions at the University of California-San Francisco, CCPH seeks to work collaboratively across sectors of higher education, communities and disciplines to achieve successful community–campus partnerships. Promoting service–learning as a core component of health professions education is one of CCPH's four strategies for fulfilling its mission.

An overview of service–learning: opportunities for nursing education

What health professions schools and their educators face today is a new paradigm of training, educating and providing care in the community. Service-learning, while relatively new to nursing education, has shown promise as an effective tool for responding to this new paradigm. Recently, service–learning has gained greater recognition in the nursing community as a curricular strategy for preparing students for their roles as nurses and citizens, changing the way faculty teach, changing the way nursing education programmes relate to their communities, enabling community organisations and community members to play significant roles in how nurses are educated, and enhancing community capacity to improve health.

Taking common elements from over 100 service–learning defini-

tions, CCPH defines service–learning as a structured learning experience that combines community service with explicit learning objectives, preparation and reflection. Students involved in service–learning
are expected not only to provide direct community service but also to
learn about the context in which the service is provided, the connection
between the service and their academic coursework, and their roles as
citizens (Jacoby, 1996; Seifer, 1997). Service–learning is a form of
experiential education that:

- is developed, implemented and evaluated in collaboration with the
  community
- responds to community identified concerns
- attempts to balance the service that is provided and the learning that
  takes place
- enhances the curriculum by extending learning beyond the classroom and allowing students to apply what they've learned to real-
  world situations
- provides opportunities for critical reflection.

Service–learning is significantly different from traditional clinical
education and is encouraged in the early years of a student's course of
study. Service–learning is not meant to replace clinical education, but
rather complement the clinical experience by:

- offering a balance between service and learning objectives
- placing an emphasis on reciprocal learning
- focusing on the development of citizenship skills
- addressing community identified concerns
- involving community in the service–learning design and implementation.

Several of the schools participating in the HPSISN programme have
designed service–learning activities in non-clinical settings such as
elementary schools, churches, neighbourhood centres and homeless
shelters.

An examination of a HPSISN grantee, the Virginia Commonwealth
University (VCU) School of Nursing, will provide insight into the
service–learning activities within a nursing school, including community partnership building, student and faculty development, reflection
strategies, and evaluation. The overview of this programme will
conclude with a series of lessons learned by the VCU team.

Service–learning in nursing education: the Linkages programme at Virginia Commonwealth University

The Virginia Commonwealth University Service–Learning Perspective

Virginia Commonwealth University is a large, urban, research institution with two campuses – a health science campus and an academic campus – in Richmond, Virginia. It considers service–learning as the vehicle to bring faculty, students and communities together. This active learning strategy that involves all the players in the university and community benefits all. It is defined as:

> the coming together of these two notions: our innate desire to contribute and our desire to learn as human beings.
> (Sigmon, quoted in Seifer, 1997).

The 'service' and 'learning' occurs in both community and campus settings. It requires that faculty and students reflect on the experiences that the community teaches. Course and curricula objectives are met not through faculty determined experiences but by faculty, student and community agreed upon experiences. Traditional clinical experiences are dramatically modified to include the perspectives and needs of all and not just the learning needs of students.

An overview of the Linkages programme goals and objectives

The overall goal of Linkages was to develop programmes of service–learning across the health professional schools at VCU. This was to be accomplished through a model of service–learning for students in required courses and extra-curricular experiences. Additional objectives were to document the impact of the service–learning programme on nursing students, faculty and community and on the health status of clients served, and to institutionalise service–learning. The objectives of the Linkages project were accomplished as faculty relinquished some control over placement of students in the community by including community agencies in the decision making about experiences. This shift in thinking occurred as faculty approached the community agencies to learn, not just to teach. The result is that both faculty and student realised the value of understanding differing views of life and community. Virginia Commonwealth University has modern class-rooms, extensive educational technology and a hospital which is ranked among the best in the nation, but priceless education is achieved outside these boundaries. Linkages required a shift in attitude towards collaboration across schools and with the community.

Discovery and application of knowledge by students in the Linkages programme

The impact of service–learning on students, faculty and community has been measured, but it is the reports of students that show the value of this shift in education. They reported that their perspective of the world was altered. The first group of undergraduate nursing students to participate in Linkages have graduated. Twenty-six elected service–learning in their first nursing course, one clinical group served as a pilot in their junior psychiatric nursing practicum, and all 80 developed service–learning projects in their senior level community health nur-sing course. Two subsequent classes have entered since the project began and are enrolled in service–learning courses. Service-learning remains an elective experience in the first nursing course; both psychiatric nursing and community health nursing courses have required service–learning components. A total of 240 nursing students have been a part of Linkages during the last three years. Student impact is measured by the hours of service that students provide, logs that students have kept, feedback from small group reflection sessions, and evaluation of the content and quality of student projects completed for community agencies.

Publications of VCU and community agencies highlight the contri-butions that students and the implementation of the service learning philosophy make to the people of the community. Student logs and reflection sessions are rich sources for learning about the impact that service learning has on the students. One student worked in an agency that provides parenting classes for teenage mothers, and another worked as a mentor for a teenage mother, both talked about being in the 'colour minority', a new experience for white students, and both discussed their own anxieties about wanting to be liked by the African-American teenagers. Their strongest responses were that they wanted the teenagers to have the same advantages they themselves had enjoyed. They talked about the teenagers' poverty, their broken appointments, and the violence that was a frequent part of their lives. Both students questioned whether or not they actually helped, but both commented on learning about a culture different from their own. Another student discovered that residents of a traditional shelter programme need clean socks and good foot care, and discovered that 'getting back on their feet' had multiple meanings, not the least of which was the basic physical need before the more complex needs of finding steady employment and a home could be met. Another saw the long-term commitment of a loving faith community who sponsored a family for five years as the family sought independence through home ownership. They carry the stories of these people with them into their more traditional nursing experience. Their perspectives of the world changed and they changed their faculty.

Community partnership building in the Linkages programme

Connections to community agencies take time and often personal connections in development. After three years trying to connect students with clients in the community who have HIV, the connection finally worked. Eight students worked in a free clinic's HIV Buddy Programme. The students faced their fears and stereotypes as they met their 'buddies' and established caring relationships with them. They sometimes encountered death, but learned about innate human dignity. One student listened as her buddy described fractured family relationships, but was amazed at his hope. Another met an elderly buddy, who opened her eyes to her own prejudices by his kindness and anticipation of her visits, but who ironically, tried to engage her in a conversation about his own racial biases. At the end of experiences student logs frequently include *'thank you for giving me this wonderful opportunity'*.

Reflection activities in the Linkages programme

Reflection is an integral activity of the service–learning experience. The reflection component assists students to see the demands placed on the community agencies, and not just their own learning needs. This has helped students be less judgemental in their evaluation of the community experience. Community agency staff and Linkages advisory board members serve as facilitators of the reflection sessions. The inclusion of community members in the reflection sessions assures that student's observations and responses are validated from not only the university perspective but also that of the community.

Challenges in the Linkages programme

The Linkages programme has been challenged by issues of time: curriculum revisions can lead to delays in implementing service–learning goals and faculty research reduces the time available for service and community outreach. Larson (1995) cited barriers as costs, faculty attitudes and scheduling difficulties that were barriers in this project as well. Having administrative support at VCU for service learning has institutionalised Linkages in the School of Nursing, and limited additional time demands on faculty.

Lessons learned in the Linkages programme

Throughout the duration of the service–learning activities at VCU, the team has learned important lessons for the ongoing implementation and sustainability of current efforts, including the following:

Institutional Leadership Matters: Leadership plays an important role in supporting service–learning efforts. The grant funding of the HPSISN programme supported a health sciences campus service–learning coordinator. This faculty member served as the support for other faculty who wanted to implement service–learning but lacked the knowledge of the community or felt that they did not have the time to commit to developing community placements. The service–learning coordinator worked with faculty from across the schools. The Provost established the Office of Community Programs, which was charged with the development and the support of service–learning courses in the general education component of undergraduate education. Through the collaboration of the Linkages programme and the Office of Community Programs, an annual Service-Learning Institute and a Service-Learning Associates Program were established.

It is not just the administrative leadership and the infrastructure that make new innovations work but also the leadership of individual faculty as they work to change their courses. For example, attendance at the university-wide Service-Learning Institute prompted a School of Pharmacy faculty member to learn about service–learning. He enrolled in the Service-Learning Associates Program. This year-long programme brings faculty together twice a month to develop service–learning courses and to study teaching methods which include community-based collaboration. The Linkages coordinator assisted him in integrating service–learning into his course and provided course consultation and evaluation materials for this pharmacy course.

Faculty Development in Service-Learning is Essential: Faculty development has played an important role in sustaining the service–learning programme. Prior to receiving the HPSISN grant, no faculty or students in the School of Nursing, or at VCU for that matter, had engaged in service–learning. The HPSISN grant and the link to the Office of Community Programs created the momentum necessary to move forward. At first, faculty were unsure of how this new approach service learning was different from the traditional 'clinical lab'. Community partners clearly identified the difference. The term 'partner' would have to be accepted if the project was to succeed. Faculty had to send students out with the instructions to listen and do what those community partners said they needed done, and: '*we'll make sense of it somehow back here at school*'. The Linkages coordinator was key to educating faculty and facilitating their work. The faculty reward and advancement in this setting traditionally comes from a formal programme of research, not service. Faculty who include service must merge it with their scholarship and teaching. Since the environment of a major research state university supports the tripartite mission of teaching, research and service, faculty are expected to maintain accomplishment in all three areas. Linkages experiences have enabled us to develop the scholarship activities of discovery, integration, teaching and application.

Faculty and students have presented posters and workshops at national and regional conferences on service–learning course development, community partnerships with the family service agency, and service–learning evaluation and implementation. Faculty work with students to develop a class mission, to help them actualise it, and have presented this work at a national nursing education conference. Service-learning developed on VCU's academic campus at the same time that the Linkages programme was funded. The university's strategic plan focused on service to the community. The Director of the Office of Community Programs took the leadership in developing a university-wide strategy. She organised the first university-sponsored conference on service–learning, inviting community partners as well as faculty and students from across the university. With the support of the Linkages project, the Faculty Service Associates programme developed, in which funding was available to help faculty implement service–learning courses. Six Service Associate faculty taught seven courses in 1997 and seven faculty have been selected as Service Associates in 1998. Collaboration with the Linkages was important in creating the nucleus for growth, and for the institutionalisation of service–learning.

Evaluation and Demonstration of Programme Success is Important: Measuring the outcomes of educational changes is vital to sustain the change within the curriculum. The service–learning coordinator developed an instrument for course faculty use in evaluating student learning. Based on this a formal instrument was developed by the VCU Office of Community Programs staff and data were collected from across the university on student learning in service–learning courses. Instruments were distributed not only to students, but also to community partners.

Student response rate was good, and community partner response rate was also good. Faculty evaluations are through the Service-Learning Associates Program. Faculty commitment was measured by the degree of integration of service–learning into curricular and professional pursuits. Participation has been centred primarily in the School of Nursing Department of Integrative Systems, where the nursing specialties of community health, nursing systems and psychiatric nursing are taught. The Integrative Systems department in the School of Nursing (SON) has revised its mission to assure that faculty and students study how various systems interface, and how the concept of 'community' can stimulate service as an ongoing health professional responsibility.

The teaching model in the SON has come under serious scrutiny for the past year and the role of collateral (non-tenure) track faculty is emerging as a dynamic one, in which scholarship efforts can take directions that do not normally reward those in tenure tracks. The collateral faculty in the SON have sustained the work of Linkages, and have begun to disseminate their service scholarship through presentations and publications.

Drawing upon the successes of the service–learning programme such as VCU may contribute to other's understanding about the benefits of this methodology. The following section describes many of the demonstrative benefits of service–learning learned through the experiences of all HPSISN sites, and affirms what has been learned at VCU.

The impact of service–learning in health professions education: lessons from the Health Professions Schools in Service to the Nation sites

Findings from the two-year evaluation of the HPSISN sites point to demonstrative benefits of service–learning to the overall partnership and its stakeholders, including the institution, student, faculty and community (Gelmon *et al.*, 1998). These benefits are as follows.

- **The nature of the overall community–campus partnership is strengthened**. The HPSISN programme had a strong impact on partnerships where the community partners were incorporated into the 'teaching, learning and assessment team' and were seen as individuals contributing to the student's learning goals. Community partners also value contributing as 'co-teachers' in the student's learning process. At VCU, the community partners are involved in the reflection sessions to ensure a balanced perspective of the student's learning in the community.
- **The preparation of students as change agents is improved**. Students were eager to be out of the classroom and engaged in activities that:

    had a clear purpose and gave them a sense of responsibility and leadership.

    Students valued the connection between the course content and community experience, and pointed to their developed skills in sensitivity towards diverse populations and awareness of community needs and issues. These conclusions are validated by VCU's students who participated in the HIV Buddy programme and became more sensitive to the issues facing this population.
- **Faculty awareness of community issues is improved**. Faculty gained a greater sense of the scope of community health needs and the resources to address them. Faculty involvement and their frequent on-going communication with the community partners were the most important elements in the sustainability of the partnership. At VCU, the institution hired a service–learning coordinator to work with faculty from across the schools. The coordinator ensured effective communication with community partners and streamlined activities.
- **Institutional image is positive**. Leadership support of service–learning strengthened positive perceptions by the community of the campus

culture. Service-learning efforts supported by the institution influenced the breakdown of the 'ivory tower' and inaccessible campus image. Establishing an Office of Community Programs at VCU provided a link between the community and the institution. Before the establishment of this office, the community would have had less of an entry into the culture of the institution.

* **Services received by community are expanded.** Through service–learning activities community partners became more aware of the resources of the institution, and appreciated the institution's recognition of the community's resources. Community partners recognised they were receiving services that would not have been possible without the service–learning activities. Publications of VCU and the community agencies highlight the contributions of the student and the services they provided.

Emphasising the benefits of service–learning and the value of community engagement may be considered the first step in preparing for change within the curriculum, the culture of the institutional community, and the broader community as a whole. What can nursing educators do to prepare for changes within the curriculum through service–learning? The following section provides a series of national and local recommendations that will assist nursing educators in their efforts.

What can nurse educators do? Recommendations for the future

The following series of recommendations provide some insight into the leadership role nursing educators can play in fostering renewed commitment in the community, and developing more meaningful community–campus partnerships through service–learning.

International and national

Become a member of CCPH. By becoming a member of CCPH, nursing educators will join a multidisciplinary membership network comprised of community and health professions leaders. Membership includes access to a worldwide membership network, an electronic discussion list, specialist publications, training, conferences and much more. A visit to the CCPH website will provide more information about membership services and the organisation's history. To find out more about CCPH, its programmes and membership opportunities, please contact Jennet Lee, Program Assistant, by phone: 415/476-7081, by email: ccph@itsa.ucsf.edu, or visit our website at http://futurehealth.ucsf.edu/ccph.html

Learn from the HPSISN sites and the teams participating in the Partners in Caring and Community: Service-Learning in Nursing Education Program. The HPSISN sites have direct experience in integrating service–learning into multidisciplinary coursework. In addition, the Partners in Caring and Community programme, an activity of CCPH and supported by the Helene Fuld Health Trust, supports ten teams of nursing faculty, students and community partners in their service–learning activities. More information about the HPSISN sites and the Partners in Caring and Community nursing teams can be obtained by contacting CCPH. The lessons learned from the HPSISN sites have contributed to the development of the CCPH resource guide *Developing Community-Responsive Models in Health Professions Education* and the HPSISN evaluation report and assessment tool workbook.

In the US

Adopt and advocate for the integration of the Pew Health Professions Commission recommendations and core competencies. Health professions schools that support service–learning in course-based activities are streets ahead of other schools in adopting the Pew Health Professions Commission core competencies for the effective practice in today's workforce. Service-learning and community service are potential tools for building community–campus partnerships and effective leaders for tomorrow's workforce. A copy of the Commission's fourth report *Recreating Health Professional Practice for a New Century* can be obtained from CCPH.

Local/institutional level

Build upon existing community relations. Perhaps a first step in integrating service–learning into coursework is to build upon existing community relations with the local school of nursing. Faculty may already be involved as volunteers at a local agency or on the board of directors of a community organisation. Drawing upon community connections provides a strong foundation for service–learning.

Identify 'faculty service enclaves' in the department or school (Burack, 1998). The chances are that there are 'invisible' groups of faculty within the nursing school or department who are participating in community service activities. Through the identification of faculty involved in these activities, faculty will expand their support network and resources. Within these enclaves, Burack's research (1998) demonstrates that:

> . . . *individuals operated collaboratively, oriented toward a common project or goal. They shared characteristics that enabled them to be effective . . . Ultimately, they were much more effective in addressing community and institutional issues as a collective than they were when working individually.*

Develop other faculty champions. While there are some notable faculty in each school or department known for their efforts in service–learning, it is important for these faculty to develop other champions for the future growth and sustainability of service–learning. One nursing faculty who attended the CCPH faculty institute indicated:

> *People who are comfortable on campus are hard to change. They are quite happy having me take their students out into the community, rather than doing it themselves.*

Helping to develop future champions is also a meaningful way of sharing expertise and promoting a sense of collaboration.

Conclusion

Service-learning as an educational methodology shows strong potential for improving nursing education and the future of the nursing profession. While the authors have provided a series of recommendations and suggestions for the development of service–learning in nursing education, more can be done. As the healthcare system continues to evolve in the US, nursing leaders are in an excellent position to further develop community–campus partnerships through service–learning. Student education and the health of communities depend upon this happening.

References

Burack C (1998) Strengthening and sustaining faculty professional service. In: D Butler and M Hawley (eds) *Journal of Public Service and Outreach: The Changing Campus Culture*. Volume 3, Number 2. Office of the Vice President for Public Service and Outreach at the University of Georgia, Athens.

Gelmon S, Holland B and Shinnamon A (1998) *Health Professions Schools in Service to the Nation: Final Evaluation Report*. Community-Campus Partnerships for Health, San Francisco.

Jacoby B (ed) (1996) *Service-Learning in Higher Education. Concepts and Practices*. Jossey-Bass, San Francisco.

Larson EL (1995) New rules for the game: interdisciplinary education for health professionals. *Nursing Outlook* **43**(4): 180–5.

O'Neil EH (1998) *Pew Health Professions Commission. Recreating Health Professional Practice for a New Century*. Center for the Health Professions, UCSF, San Francisco

Seifer S (1997) *Overcoming a Century of Town-Gown Relations: Redefining Relationships Between Communities and Academic Health Centers. Expanding Boundaries: Service and Learning*. Corporation for National Service, Washington.

Seifer SD and Connors KM (1997) *Community-Campus Partnerships for Health. A Guide for Developing Community-Responsive Models in Health Professions Education*. Center for the Health Professions, University of California, San Francisco.

Further reading

Anderson C (1994) Nursing faculty: Who are they, what do they do, and what challenges do they face? In: J McCloskey and H Grace (eds) *Current Issues in Nursing* (4e). Mosby, St Louis.

Boyer E (1990) *Scholarship Reconsidered*. Carnegie Foundation for the Advancement of Teaching. Princeton, NJ.

Connors K *et al.* (1996) Interdisciplinary collaboration in service learning: lessons learned from the health professions. *Michigan Journal of Community Service Learning* **Fall**.

Farley S (1997) Developing professional–community partnerships. In: J McCloskey and H Grace (eds) *Current Issues in Nursing* (5e). Mosby, St Louis.

Henry JK (1997) Community nursing centers: models of nurse managed care. *JOGNN* **26**(2): 224–8.

Holland B and Gelmon S (1999) The state of the engaged campus. *American Association of Higher Education Bulletin*. In press.

Honnet EP and Poulsen SJ (1989). Principles of good practice for combining service and learning (Special Report). *The Wingspread Journal*. The Johnson Foundation Inc, Racine, WI.

Lynton EA (1995) *Making the Case for Professional Service*. American Association for Higher Education, Washington DC.

Maurana C and Goldenberg K (1996) A successful academic–community partnership to improve the public's health. *Academic Medicine* **71**(5).

Rice RE (1991) The new American scholar: scholarship and the purposes of the University. *Metropolitan Universities* **Spring**: 7–18.

Richards R (1996) *Building Partnerships: Educating Health Professionals for the Communities They Serve*. Jossey-Bass, San Francisco, CA.

Seifer S (1993) Service learning: community–campus partnerships in health professions education. *Academic Medicine* **73**(3).

Seifer SD, Mutha S and Connors KM (1996). Service learning in health professions education: barriers, facilitators, and strategies for success. In: *Expanding Boundaries: Serving and Learning*. Corporation for National Service, New York.

Siegler EL and Whitney FW (1994) What is collaboration? In: EL Siegler and FW Whitney (eds) *Nurse–Physician Collaboration*. Springer Publishing Co, New York.

Australia

Healthcare, health policy and nursing

Sally Borbasi and Alan Pearson

The successful development of Australia is linked with the adaptation of new settlers to life in rural and remote locations in a sparsely populated country extending over a huge land mass. Historically, the need for adaptation in rural and remote areas was greater than in the eastern coastal cities as the rural settlers' lives depended on their capacity to adapt rapidly to the isolation. The image of the self-reliant, independent and democratic Australian was created soon after the first settlement and was a reference to the rural population, rather than the people who had settled in the cities.

More than two-thirds of the population of approximately 18 million reside in large towns and cities located on the coastal fringes of Australia's large land mass. Most of the remaining population – comprising of both indigenous people and rural people descended from a wide range of cultures – generally have access to services based on an urban model of healthcare at a much lower level in terms of resources. A smaller number of people residing in remote areas are served by remote area nurses supported by Australia's Royal Flying Doctor Service.

While the introduction of transport and communication links means that rural people are no longer isolated as they were during early settlement, there is still a distinctive difference between metropolitan and rural areas. For example, rural areas in Australia have fewer people born overseas than do the major capital cities, suggesting that the trend which began with early settlement has continued into the 1990s (Australian Bureau of Statistics, 1990). Rural people, therefore, are more likely to be Australian born than those in metropolitan areas. This means that while there are few people from a non-English speaking background (in comparison to the capital cities), those from this background who do settle in rural areas are likely to have fewer services available to meet their different cultural needs.

Public health

Until the beginning of the 20th century, infectious diseases such as tuberculosis, smallpox, typhoid and cholera were the major causes of death but these became much less of a threat to health and life amongst non-Aboriginal Australians as a result of improvements in sanitation, the introduction of enlightened public health laws and the increase in the number of public health workers (Waring Roreden and McLennan, 1992). In the non-Aboriginal population, life expectancy has increased considerably and the major causes of death are now cardiovascular disease, carcinoma and accidents. Wass (1994) suggests that Australia '. . . is now regarded as one of the healthiest countries in the world'. However, major inequalities exist in health, with some groups having considerably poorer health status than others. Most notable is the health of Aboriginal people, whose health status has been described as similar to that of the peoples of the developing world.

Indigenous Australians are more likely to smoke tobacco, be non-participative in leisure-time physical activity and be obese. Other statistics show them to die from cardiovascular disease at twice the rate of other Australians and to be far more prone to diseases such as rheumatic fever and type II diabetes than other Australians. In 1995, compared with 3% of other Australians, 8% of Indigenous Australians drank alcohol at harmful levels (AIHW, 1999). Petrol sniffing among the young is an area of increasing concern.

Health policy

The Australian healthcare system has been described as 'the product of a diverse range of economic, social, technological, legal, constitutional and political factors, some of which are unique to Australia' (Palmer, and Short, 1994). External influences stem from countries such as Canada, Great Britain and the United States. The basis of the Australian healthcare system is Medicare; a centrally administered form of universal tax-funded health insurance that has taken shape since 1972 when it was first introduced by the Australian Labour Party (as Medibank) (Short et al., 1993). Under this system 'free' hospital care is available to all Australians. For those who choose it and can afford it, private health insurance offers an alternative. Whereas each state and territory is primarily responsible for the provision of services, the major responsibility for funding and setting policy for the Medicare system lies with the Commonwealth government (Malko, 1997). This is a source of constant conflict between the federal and state governments as the cost of providing a health service escalates.

As in other developed nations, healthcare is now a huge and complex industry. Billions of dollars per year are expended on the nation's health, approximating 9% of GDP (Malko, 1997). Increasing cost is manifested in constraints or limitations on the provision of an equitable system. In accordance with the coalition government's microeconomic reform efforts are underway to move to a market model of healthcare (Malko, 1997). Efforts to increase revenue for Medicare have meant individuals pay a levy on their incomes. While this can be viewed as a fairly low percentage, it rises each year (Daniel, 1998). More recently in order to persuade higher income earners to invest in private health insurance, the government has offered a rebate incentive and those who earn over a certain threshold who do not have private insurance are required to pay a higher Medicare levy. In the states and territories, public hospital spending is capped and most are now funded according to diagnostic related groups (DRGs) and casemix. Benchmarking and clinical pathway implementation is increasing together with patient classification systems. According to economists, one of the major drawbacks of the Australian healthcare system is that fee for service in terms of other medical services outside hospitals is not capped.

Health services generally can be defined as having two major targets comprising the population and the environment (Malko, 1997). As in other parts of the western world, the locus of care is shifting from the acute care sector to the community. Ambulatory care, day surgery, hospitals in the home, and co-ordinated (continuous) community care through regional demonstration units are all developments designed to reduce/shift the financial burden of ill health. For nurses these changes offer opportunities as never before and scope of practice is an area under increasing review. Nurses in New South Wales, for example, have recently been successful in legislating for a nurse practitioner role and there are moves for similar legislation in other States. In South Australia the role of the nurse practitioner and the issue of credentialling are topical issues and the profession has recently secured clinical admitting privileges for advanced practice nurses and midwives to acute-care facilities. Evidence-based nursing practice has also emerged as an area of contemporary interest to nurses. This has led to the establishment of The Joanna Briggs Institute for Evidence-Based Nursing (JBIEBN) based at the Royal Adelaide Hospital in South Australia. This institute contributes to the evidence base for nursing through the systematic review of research, the dissemination of information for the development of practice guidelines, primary research and the promotion of evidence-based practice.

Nursing

In common with a number of other countries, the development of healthcare in Australia has relied heavily on the work of nurses. This is particularly true of rural nurses. In the late 19th century and the first half of the 20th century, nurses provided extensive healthcare services without any readily available access to medical or allied health personnel, other than via radio or other form of telecommunication. For the most part, the services provided by nurses were highly regarded by rural people, and the health status of these people has steadily increased.

Nursing education and practice in Australia, as in other parts of the world, is in the midst of rapid change. Pressure for increased opportunities for higher nursing education and for changes in the organisation of nursing practice are part of wider demands. Such demands include the recognition of nursing as central to the reorganisation of health services to reflect both client-centred care and effective and efficient resource management at local, state and federal level.

With regard to nursing education, Australia was part of the wordwide trend that reorientated nursing education in the 1980s. In Northern Europe, North America and Australia nursing education relocated itself from the vocational to the higher education sector. Following a long process of lobbying by Australian nurses, the federal government announced in 1984 that nursing education would be totally transferred to the advanced education sector by 1993. (The advanced education sector was, at that time, separate to the university system and focused on vocational education at the Bachelor and Master degree level.) Subsequent to this momentous decision, one university school of nursing was established in 1987, which offered a PhD programme in nursing in that year, and the advanced education sector was merged with the university sector to form a Unified National Higher Education System with university status conferred on most institutions by 1990 (Commonwealth of Australia, 1994).

The only route to registration as a nurse in all states and territories of Australia is through the acquisition of a Bachelor of Nursing degree from a recognised university. Following on from this important development for nursing, postgraduate diploma programmes in clinical specialties, Master's degrees in nursing and PhD degrees in nursing have proliferated and there is a rapidly increasing pool of Master's degree graduates seeking entry to PhD programmes in university schools of nursing. While this is indeed a source of great pride to Australian nurses, it is becoming increasingly clear to some nursing leaders that PhD preparation focuses on independent research activity and the education of academics and career researchers. Thus, contemporary nursing in Australia (and elsewhere!) is characterised by a flourishing academic role within the universities, but such growth and development is not matched in nursing practice or health service delivery.

The need to create opportunities for those nurses in practice and service leadership (whose interests do not coincide with those of academics and scholarly researchers) to pursue higher degree studies to the doctoral level is becoming increasingly evident. As a result, two Australian nursing schools (The University of Adelaide and La Trobe University – both situated in leading research universities) have developed professional doctorates, the Doctor of Nursing degree, with a clear focus on professional practice. Whilst North America has a history of offering Doctor of Nursing Science degrees, and both Britain and North America offer PhD degrees for nurses, the Australian Nursing Doctorate is different. It is a professional doctorate requiring professional practice to be underpinned rather than led by research, which equips flexible nurses to help lead colleagues into an uncertain future.

More details about the Australian Nursing Doctorate and the issues it raises will be provided in the final chapter of this book. This next section focuses on two aspects of nursing practice in Australia; the extended role of rural nurses (Chapter Seven), and the advanced role of nurse practitioners (Chapter Eight).

References

Australian Insititute of Health and Welfare (AIHW) and Heart Foundation of Australia (HFA) (1999) *Heart, Stroke and Vascular Diseases: Australian Facts.* AIHW and the HFA, Canberra.

ABS (1990) *Australian National Accounts Input–Output Tables, 1986–1987.* Australian Bureau of Statistics, Canberra.

Commonwealth of Australia (1994) *A Unified National Higher Education System.* Commonwealth of Australia, Canberra.

Daniel A (1998) The politics of health: medicine versus the state. In: G Lupton and J Najman (eds) *Sociology of Health and Illness: Australian Readings* (2e). University of Queensland, Brisbane.

Malko C (1997) The environment of healthcare in Australia. In: M Courtney (ed) *Financial Management in Health Services*. MacLennan & Petty, Sydney.

Palmer G and Short S (1994) *Health Care & Public Policy: An Australian Analysis* (2e). MacMillan Education, Melbourne.

Short S, Sharman E and Speedy S (1993) *Sociology for Nurses: An Australian Introduction*. MacMillan Education, Melbourne.

Waring Roreden J and McLennan J (1992) *Community Health Nursing. Theory and Practice*. Harcourt Brace Jovanovitch, Sydney.

Wass A (1994) *Promoting Health. The Primary Health Care Approach*. Harcourt Brace Jovanovitch, Sydney.

CHAPTER SEVEN

Serving the community: the rural general practice nurse

Alan Pearson, Denise Hegney and Pauline Donnelly

> *it is entirely appropriate to extend nurses' roles in remote and rural contexts to improve nursing, in its purest sense, by building up nursing knowledge and equipping nurses to provide nursing expertise for those who need it. Such a view is acceptable if the purpose of nursing is to meet the needs of the society which it serves.* (Pearson, 1993)

In this chapter we focus on the health policy implications of Australia's sparsely populated rural areas. We do so to highlight how health policy imperatives drive changes in nursing and, conversely, create openings for nurses to shape policy in their response to the needs of the community for healthcare.

The chapter draws largely on an extensive study carried out by two of us on the role of the rural nurse in Australia (Hegney *et al.*, 1998).[1] While it is acknowledged that there may be similarities between Australia and other developed countries, such as Canada and the United States, there is no reference to publications from sources other than Australia.

[1] This study, *The Role and Function of the Rural Nurse in Australia* was supported by a Commonwealth Department of Health and Family Services, Rural Health Support, Education and Training Grant (Grant No. 245 – The Role and Function of the Rural Nurse, and Grant No. 341 – A National Investigation and Support Project for Australian Rural Nurses).

Rural nursing: responding to and driving policy

The exponential growth in medical science, the increasing sophistication of health service consumers' knowledge, and the proliferation of medical specialists in the latter half of the 20th century have all contributed to the desire of rural people to have access to medical practitioners and health specialists, and to the increasing ambiguity surrounding the legitimate role of the rural nurse. Organised rural nursing in Australia began when the first non-indigenous people moved into rural areas. After white settlement both men and women, often untrained, provided nursing to rural communities on a largely ad-hoc basis. It was not until the 'bush nursing' services were established and the so-called 'Nightingale' reforms became well regarded that nursing services (as we know them today) became gendered and began to provide health service delivery to rural communities. Thus, since early white settlement, nurses have played a central role in ensuring that rural communities (regardless of size) have access to a health service. Although some notable medical practitioners feature highly in the often romanticised histories of rural life in Australia, such figures were rare in the first 140 years of European settlement and the invisibility of rural nurses in Australian literature says much more about Australia's attitudes to nursing than it does about the reality of the evolution of rural healthcare.

Primary healthcare in Australia

Primary healthcare can be a level of service provision and an approach to healthcare. As a level of service provision, it is the first level of contact with the health system for a resident. Primary healthcare is also a healthcare policy approach which (Palmer and Short, 1994, quoted in Hegney *et al.*, 1998):

> *seeks to extend healthcare beyond therapeutic care to health promotion, which is given low priority in our present illness-orientated care system.*

Nurses who speak about primary healthcare delivery state that: '*rural nurses are often the only available health professional to serve the immediate needs of the local community*' (Spencer, 1994). These nurses are also recognised as a resource for information and support with regard to a wide range of health-related issues (Hart *et al.*, 1992, quoted in Hegney *et al.*, 1998). They are seen to function as primary care providers and health educators, without direct medical support (Dunning *et al.*, 1994).

Nursing researchers, nursing academics and community health nurses frequently discuss the role of primary healthcare as a model of service delivery in the literature. The literature in this area largely relates to how nurses should provide a primary healthcare approach, or are reports from nurses who have provided a service which they believe has a primary healthcare approach.

The type of service most frequently described is Women's Health, and the achievement of the best possible healthcare for rural women. For example, Fuller and Gartley (1993) describe a Women's Health Service which has a primary healthcare focus as it involves community development based on social justice strategies and is multidisciplinary. In this context the term multidisciplinary is not used as it appears in the policy documents, rather there is a recognition that Women's Health Services need to have the involvement of all (including the community) to ensure that health status is improved.

Livingstone-Vail (1994) notes that there are barriers to primary healthcare which have yet to be overcome. She asserts that inter-disciplinary tensions, poor communication, remuneration mechanisms based on fee-for-service, and lack of awareness of primary healthcare continue to prevent the successful adoption of this model. In addition, it has been suggested that successful prevention programmes work on community involvement and commitment, and cannot be measured on throughput, adjusted daily bed average or cost per bed/day: the (easy to measure) performance indicators favoured by politicians and health service planners and managers.

The extended role of rural nurses

Rural Australians are not one homogeneous group – rather, they live in settlements which are diverse in their economic base, activities and cultural composition. It is this diversity in rural communities which determines the scope of rural nursing practice. Rural nursing is said to be different to metropolitan and remote area nursing. One of the distinguishing factors identified in the literature is the generalist role of rural nurses who work in small rural health service, district and community nursing centres. This role is often described as 'extended', 'expanded' or 'multi-skilled'.

The debate surrounding the extended practice role of rural nurses is limited to those nurses who work in small rural hospitals (where there is no full-time medical officer and few allied health professionals); the district nurse (who provides an illness service); the community health nurse (who provides a preventative service); and nurses who work in the more sparsely settled areas in nursing posts (which may have a staff of one or more nurses).

Nurses who work in small rural hospitals, district and community nursing and nursing posts are required to have a broad range of knowledge and skills, many of which are not traditionally those of nursing. In these smaller health services, it is feasible that a nurse would utilise knowledge and skills related to midwifery, accident and emergency, paediatrics, medical nursing, surgical nursing and operating theatres in any one shift. In addition to nursing practice, the nurse may work as a pharmacist (dispensing medication from the hospital pharmacy), a radiographer (taking X-rays), a medical practitioner (assessment and diagnosis of patients, admission and discharge of patients, intubation and other forms of emergency care), a physiotherapist, an occupational therapist, and a social worker (counselling and other social work skills).

Nurses who are employed in the larger health services in rural areas have a scope of practice which is similar to that of nurses in metropolitan areas. The larger centres usually have resident medical officers, specialists and a range of allied health professionals and other support services. In addition, nurses who work in the base or provincial hospitals are more likely to work in one area, for example midwifery, paediatrics, medical nursing or intensive care. These nurses rarely have the same need for generalist knowledge and skills and few work in an extended practice role.

Community nurses and district nurses who work in small rural communities are seen as requiring a broader range of skills than those who work in larger settings (Lampshire and Rolfe, 1991). It is the lack of support services which influences the scope of these nurses' practice.

The need for rural nurses to have a broad range of knowledge and skills was first mentioned by Staunton (1991), who noted that: *'nurses often diagnose, treat and are surrogate doctor'*. Nurses often make the initial assessment of patients and decide whether to call the medical officer, send the patient home or admit them to hospital. This function (the admission and discharge of patients) is outside the nurse's role: '[the nurse] *must make the doctor come to the hospital and make the decision'* (Staunton, 1991). Rural nurses have a generalist role (though this term is not used in the discourse of rural nursing) which is not recognised within the nursing profession as specialist in nature, as nursing specialists, like medical specialists, are known to work in one discrete area, for example, diabetes, paediatrics, midwifery or intensive care.

It has been suggested that this lack of recognition of a specialist generalist role for rural nurses has disadvantaged practitioners in many areas, such as preparation for their role, continuing education and award and career pathways (Donnelly, 1993; King, 1994). While the opportunities for career advancement are greater in capital cities (due to the size of the workforce), data from the Australian Institute of Health and Welfare (1996) suggests that the percentage of higher level clinical positions does not vary significantly between locations. It is possible that rural nurses' perception of a lack of career pathway reflects the relative stability of the workforce and many nurses' inability to move to a more senior position in another town because of family and economic considerations.

In addition to the wide range of knowledge and skills necessary to provide competent and confident practice in rural areas, many nurses (particularly those working in small communities) are required to extend their role into the domain of medicine, pharmacy, radiography and other allied health discipline areas. The extended practice role of rural nurses has been noted and authors have also expressed the opinion that rural nurses are not adequately educationally prepared for these roles (Kreger, 1991; Pearson, 1993; King, 1994).

Extension of the nurse's role is not new to rural settings, as it was the early 'bush' nurses who provided the majority of care to rural communities prior to the expansion of the population and the resultant increase in service provision. What is, then, an extended role and how it is used in the rural nursing? Zornow (1977, cited in Pearson, 1993) saw extension as: *'elongating specific, already assumed functions to fill perceived gaps'*.

It has been suggested that the additional tasks incorporated into the nurse's role are essentially medical in nature. Both of these definitions are used to describe the need for an extended role for rural and remote area nurses. The reason given for the extended practice role of rural nurses is the need to provide a health service to a community who have been educated into a medical-specialist model of healthcare (King, 1994). Without this extended role, Kreger argues (1991), the health needs of the community would not be met:

> *Public access to medical, pharmaceutical and preventative orientated services would diminish if rural and remote area nurses adhered to existing legislation and the traditional expectations of professional relationships and practice.*

With the current reluctance of medical practitioners to work in small rural areas and the inability of health services to employ a range of allied health professionals (due to the cost), if nurses did not 'fill the gap', the service would not be provided. Therefore, extended practice roles are essential to the provision of health services in rural areas.

Despite the fact that many rural nurses have traditionally worked in this extended role, current policy usually refers to the need to be 'multi-skilled', rather than acknowledging the traditional extended role. Pearson (1993) states that the term multi-skilling is the new 'in word' for extension and expansion of healthcare providers' roles. He argues:

> It is entirely appropriate to extend nurses' roles in remote and rural contexts to improve nursing, in its purest sense, by building up nursing knowledge and equipping nurses to provide nursing expertise for those who need it. Such a view is acceptable if the purpose of nursing is to meet the needs of the society which it serves.

The majority of rural nurses are not prepared for this role either in their undergraduate education or in the scope of continuing professional and award education which has been traditionally available (King, 1994).

Analysis of the literature indicates that the issue of role extension in healthcare, and the consequent blurring of role boundaries, has largely been confined to the discipline of nursing. Hodgson (1992), however, highlights the concern of allied health professionals in rural and remote areas on the trend towards multi-skilling. Vernon (1994) has expressed the opinion that the introduction of multi-purpose health centres will increase the need for a multi-skilled nursing workforce. She argues that multi-skilling provides an exciting and new challenge for nurses, and encourages them to embrace the change. The statements on the need for a multi-skilled workforce (particularly relating to multi-purpose health centres) do not at any time acknowledge that the majority of nurses who work in small rural health services have always been 'multi-skilled'.

The majority of statements on the need for an extended nursing role relate to the need to 'fill the gaps', due to the lack of medical and allied health professionals. The extended practice role which is discussed is one of 'cure'. The arguments, therefore, appear to be based on the nurse working in an extended practice role when other services are not available, and improving the cost-effectiveness of services. In contrast, many nurses who discuss the extended practice role of rural nurses call for the legitimisation of the extended role, which they see as having a health promotion, as well as a care and cure dimension.

The shortage of medical practitioners and allied health professionals: nurses 'filling the gap'

In Australia, health services to small rural communities contain a mix of the following:

- a full-time medical general practitioner in the town
- a visiting general practitioner
- access to the Royal Flying Doctor Service (RFDS) (who provide medical clinics as well as emergency evacuations)
- visiting medical specialists (most commonly surgeons who are flown into the town)
- a full-time pharmacist in the town (who also provides a service at the hospital)
- a remote pharmacist (usually in a neighbouring town)
- varying levels of allied health services (radiographer, social worker, physiotherapist, occupational therapist)
- visiting allied health services (for example, mental health teams and aged care assessment teams)
- mobile screening vans (mammography units, women's health vans).

The extended role of the nurse varies depending on the type and number of support services available at any one time. The nurse, however, is always able to contact a medical practitioner by telephone or radio for consultation and advice. For example, nurses who work in towns where there is no medical service usually have 24-hour access to the RFDS. In other cases, where there is only one medical officer in the town and the medical officer is absent, the nurse may have to contact a medical officer in a neighbouring town. Despite this telephone availability, there is a need for nurses who work in these smaller settings to be skilled in advanced physical assessment.

The literature suggests that, where there is no general practitioner, nurses may perform X-rays, emergency care (including cannulation, suturing, defibrillation, intubation), and family planning. Nurses extend their role in medically underserviced areas and work as substitutes for other health professionals who are either not available or provide a limited service (Dunning *et al.*, 1994). Even when medical officers are available within a town, there is often: '*an arrangement which has grown over time between the medical staff and the nursing staff who work at that hospital*' (Fisher, 1993).

McDonald (1994), reporting on her study of small rural hospitals in

New South Wales, noted that the level of what she referred to as 'autonomous' practice depended on the type of management within the hospital and the medical officers who had admission rights to the hospital. She states that: *'many doctors want to be called for every patient regardless of what is wrong with them'*. Others, she noted, did not want to be called during the night except for an extreme emergency.

Improving the cost-effectiveness of services

Surprisingly there is little emphasis on the fact that nurses who work in an extended practice role save the health service money. One director of nursing, Evans (1994), has reported on his attempt to introduce an extended role for nurses at a small hospital in Narrabri, New South Wales. He states that the decision to introduce and validate an extended role was, and always must be, based on cost-effectiveness. He argues that it is more cost-effective for nurses to be able to cannulate, introduce additives to intravenous infusion, and suture, than to contact the general practitioner 'on call'. He noted that the extension of the role could mean considerable savings for health services.

The call for acceptance and legitimisation

An extended practice role with a resultant high autonomy of decision making is not new to remote area nursing in Australia, but until relatively recently, has not been discussed in relation to rural nurses' extended practice role (Dunne, 1995). Many authors have expressed the opinion that the extended role of the nurse in rural and remote areas must be legitimised (Pearson, 1993; King, 1994; Keyzer *et al.*, 1995). The authors associate the extended practice role to the introduction of a nurse practitioner model in Australia and acknowledge that not all nurses should or would wish to work at this level of autonomy of practice.

Another aspect of the extended practice role is the legality of the work, particularly relating to dispensing, prescribing and supplying medications (Kreger, 1991; King, 1994). Before discussing the specific issues which relate to legal aspects of the nurse's role, it is important to examine some aspects of autonomy in practice.

Johnstone (1992) states:

> the full legitimated status [of nurses] as autonomous profes-
> sionals remains as strong as it was during the early days of
> the emerging modern nursing professions and many (mostly
> male doctors, hospital administrators and politicians) con-
> tinue to resist and be vehemently opposed to any thought
> that nurses should take their destiny into their own hands.

Johnstone proposes that the law assumes that nurses:

- lack full rational competence and thus the capacity to be full
  professionals and to make sound independent and reasonable professional judgements
- are the natural subordinates of medical officers and as such have a
  natural duty of obedience to medical officers
- need to be controlled and supervised by medical officers.

Rural nurses have been slow to request changes in the law to reflect
their practice. This is not the case for remote area nurses who have been
lobbying, relatively unsuccessfully, for some time to have legislation
reflect their practice. Rural and remote area nurses do not have the
legitimate authority necessary to match their responsibilities as professionals and are not legally permitted to exercise *bona fide* independent
professional judgements. Those who do risk being punished for professional misconduct, interfering with the physician–patient relationship,
insubordination, or are accused of engaging in the practice of medicine.
The conflict in rural and remote areas is that on the one hand, these
nurses can have an autonomous health practitioner role (depending on
the size of the hospital), but on the other hand, there is an understanding
that they must always follow someone else's directions. Recognising
this dilemma Staunton (1991) states: *'you can't have it both ways.'*

Despite the fact that rural nurses are frequently required to function
quite independently of medical officers, and that the majority of their
nursing actions are not performed under the supervision of medical
officers, nurses find it extremely difficult to overcome the legal barriers
that have historically denied them 'freedom to nurse' (Coxhead, 1993).
Rural nurses, therefore, are working as independent agents without
official recognition (Keyzer, 1994).

Johnstone (1992) states that the law works to keep nurses in their
proper sphere and ensures that they do not invade the area of physicians' competence and authority. This is particularly the case in rural
and remote areas, where nurses are often suppressed by the patriarchal
influence of medical officers and the more dominant discourse of
medicine (King, 1994). What is urgently needed are legal changes to

legitimise the role of the nurse. Staunton (1991), however, believes that rural nurses do not need law reform. She states:

> *It is a recognition by the authorities that you are all in potentially vulnerable legal situations and that has to be addressed in a positive way.*

There is an increasing demand amongst nurses for autonomy of nursing practice regardless of their practice setting. While there is a movement for independent practice, not all nurses seek to be independent practitioners as they do not wish to be accountable for their decisions, or defend these decisions to their peers. Rural nurses, however, especially those who work in small rural hospitals, already have extensive independence of practice and some report a high level of satisfaction with their ability to work as autonomous practitioners. In fact, it is this very nature of working in small communities that attracts some nurses to this type of practice.

Evident within the literature is another side to the debate on autonomy of practice. Dawson (1992) noted that the health outcomes from nurses working in an extended practice role are not always good. She states that:

> *The guilt experienced by nurses after such episodes could be avoided if nurses were trained and licensed to perform these types of lifesaving procedures'.*

Few other authors raise issues of non-competent nursing care in rural areas, but, given the aforementioned concern regarding the lack of on-going education and training, one would suppose that some rural nurses could well be delivering care which is outdated and unsafe.

Nursing standards

As long as nurses work within the standard which is set by the profession, they do not need to concern themselves with litigation. Yet, there are two issues which are raised by the legal statements. First, it is acknowledged that rural nurses are experiencing difficulty in accessing continuing professional education, which is necessary to ensure that they are competent and confident in their practice. One would expect, therefore, that those who have not been able to access current information are not working to an accepted standard. Second, there is no agreed standard for rural nursing practice. The question remains: what is this standard and by what scope of practice criteria is it judged?

Despite the argument that a nurse working in an extended practice role is delivering nursing care, not medical care, there is no doubt that nurses who work in small rural communities are carrying out work which, in a larger centre, would be considered to be the domain of medicine or allied health (Coxhead, 1993: Evans, 1994). Despite the rhetoric of primary healthcare, it is a medical service which rural communities value the highest and, until community expectations are overcome, nurses working in small rural communities will continue to provide a predominantly medical model service.

Employers continue to employ nurses in these extended practice roles with full knowledge that the majority of them have been ill prepared for their role. Buckley and Lambert (1994) express concern over the 'double standard' which expects the practitioner to practice beyond their level of preparation with nil (or limited) professional support, no legislative support or industrial support and limited opportunities for professional development.

Rural nursing practice: legislation and nurse prescribing rights

To practice within it, rural nurses require sound knowledge of the law. The two sources of law which impact most upon rural nursing practice (in fact, all nursing practice) are common law and parliamentary or statute law (Staunton and Wyburn, 1993). Hegney *et al.* (1998) discuss research findings in both of these areas. They say that nurses are concerned about negligence (failing to provide a duty of care; providing care below the standard expected; damage as a result of this breach of duty of care; and the foreseeability of the damage of the negligent act). In addition, they are concerned about breaches of the specific legislation which covers the control and supply of poisons in their state or territory. The areas which most affect nurses in rural areas are the Schedule 4 and 8 drugs.

The Schedule 8 (S8) drugs (drugs of addiction, dangerous drugs or narcotic substances) are more closely controlled than S4 drugs in that while nurses are able to possess and supply these drugs, they can have their authority withdrawn at any time (Staunton and Wyburn, 1993). The regulations regarding S8 drugs are similar to S4 in that medical practitioners, dentists and veterinary surgeons are the only people allowed to prescribe them. In addition, the verbal orders allowed in 'an emergency' are the same as S4 drugs (Staunton and Wyburn, 1993).

Medication issues have been raised as problematic in rural nursing by NSW Health (1995) and Hegney (1995). Pearson (1993) in his paper on the extended role of the rural nurse, noted that Thornton (1988) found that respondents in their study wanted limited prescribing rights. The NSW Nurse Practitioner Report (1995) recommends that: *'the Poisons Act and the Regulations be amended to authorise nurse practitioners to write medication orders for S3 and S4 substances from a nurses' formulary'*. Conditions which are placed upon these prescribing rights are that the drugs *'be appropriate to the context of care and the speciality area of practice '*and that *'written policies and protocols/ clinical guidelines'* must be utilised and that there be a *''mechanism for ongoing evaluation to ensure safe and appropriate practice'* (NSW Health, 1995).

Recruitment and retention of health professionals in rural areas

Despite the documented shortage of allied health professionals and remote area nurses, recruitment strategies to overcome the shortfall of medical practitioners (both general practitioners and medical specialists) have dominated health policy for the past decade. All of the policy documents, as well as the majority of policy papers presented at rural conferences, discuss the shortages (caused by lack of recruitment and retention) of general practitioners in rural areas. Despite the introduction of a Rural Incentives Program (RIP) and other measures, such as locum relief and attention to anomalies in the Medicare rebates, it appears that there remains a shortage of general practitioners in rural and remote areas. One explanation for the continued shortage is that the lack of spouse employment, inadequate educational facilities for children, and cultural deprivation ensures that many medical officers do not seek to live in rural areas.

Whilst similar issues impact upon the recruitment and retention of nurses and allied health professionals, there have been no incentive schemes established for these professions, despite the fact that lack of access to education and training has been linked to recruitment and retention issues for rural nurses (Keyzer et al., 1995).

The literature suggests that recruitment and retention of nurses in rural and remote Australia is not as severe a problem as it is with medical practitioners. Hegney *et al.* (1998) quotes Lawrence, the then Federal Minister of Health, who believed that nurses were willing and *'indeed interested in working in rural communities'*. She noted, however, that there was a need for better housing, increased security (especially in remote Australia) and networking.

The inequity of ability to access incentives for rural and remote practice for nurses and allied health professionals from rural and remote areas continues.

Recruitment and retention is one factor governing job satisfaction. Others, such as professional autonomy, have been referred to earlier. A major problem for rural nurses has been their inability to practice within a broader (primary health as opposed to primary medicine) model of health service delivery. To do so they would need to work in more effective partnership with doctors. This issue is now being addressed, as shown in the case study presented below.

Case study: the rural general practice nurse

An example of the emergence of new roles in rural Australia is the general practice nurse in South Australia.

The South Australian government's Department of Human Services commenced funding a postgraduate programme for preparing general practice nurses in 1998. The one-year, full-time (or two-year, part-time) programme is offered jointly by the Department of Clinical Nursing and the Department of General Practice, both situated with the School of Medicine at the University of Adelaide, and leads to the award of Graduate Diploma in General Practice Nursing (GraDipGen-PractNurs).

The programme content area includes: epidemiology, public health, primary healthcare, nursing practice, health surveillance, health promotion, health screening, the management of chronic health conditions and the diagnosis and treatment of minor illnesses and trauma. In semester one of the programme, students work alongside a medical general practitioner who acts as a clinical tutor in general practice. In semester two, students are placed in an emergency department and are required to gain proficiency in the assessment and treatment of minor trauma.

The role of one of the graduates of this programme serves to demonstrate the emergence of the rural general practice nurse.

'Margaret' is a registered nurse who completed her hospital nursing training in the 1970s in a small, rural hospital and later gained a Bachelor degree in nursing. She is married with children and has worked as a nurse-receptionist with a team of general practitioners in a small rural town in South Australia. The general practitioners with whom she works are very involved in town life and are often on-call to provide medical cover to the local population. Despite a number of attempts to recruit additional partners to the practice (including the offer of a range of incentives) it has proved to be difficult to maintain a comprehensive medical service to the area and all of the partners agreed to support the secondment of nurses within the practice to a programme to extend and expand their knowledge and skills, and to increase nursing input into the operations of the practice.

The general practitioners hoped to reorganise their work by eventually establishing an on-call system of general practice nurses to receive 'firstcalls' and refer on to the on-call doctor when required. They also wanted nurses to be skilled in the ongoing continuing care of patients with long-term disabilities and illnesses; the carrying out of health screening activities, such as pap smears; the administration of immunisations; and the treatment of minor injuries and complaints, such as the suturing or treatment of minor wounds, and the removal of foreign bodies.

Having completed the GradDipGenPractNurs, Margaret no longer performs receptionist duties. She now runs four nursing clinics a week in the practice, mainly involving dressings, immunisations and investigations. The monitoring of patients over 85 years of age through regular assessments, either in the practice or on home visits, is also now her responsibility and she is awaiting the completion of the programme by one of her colleagues before working with the doctors to establish working protocols in order to commence a nurse on-call roster.

Margaret feels increasingly satisfied with her work and is of the view that her expanded role improves the overall service to patients. Not only does her input reduce the excessive workloads for doctors, but her nursing expertise enables her to emphasise health promotion when she sees patients, and her extensive local knowledge informs her interventions. There is now no perceived need in this practice to recruit additional general practitioners. The current, stable and high-functioning team have, through working with the community, identified needs and agreed on skilling staff within the team to meet these needs. Although this is still developing, the team themselves are aware of a growth in trust between Margaret and the doctors, and an increasing demand on nursing input from the community.

Conclusion

Rural practice in Australia has always operated uncomfortably in line with policies developed for densely populated urban areas. In meeting the needs of rural people, such policies and protocols have usually been modified by doctors and nurses. Policy makers, knowing this to be the case, have generally 'turned a blind eye', but have not attempted to generate policy for rural practice. Current health policy in Australia is redressing this failure to acknowledge that rural healthcare differs from urban healthcare and this presents a wide range of opportunities for nursing.

References

Australian Institute of Health and Welfare (1996) National Nurse Labourforce Collection – 1993. Unpublished data.

Buckley P and Lambert EL (1994) *Rural health – a practice affirmation model*. Paper presented at the Windmills, Wisdom and Wonderment Conference of the Association for Australian Rural Nurses Inc., Roseworthy.

Coxhead J (1993) United we stand – divided we fall. *The Australian Journal of Rural Health* **1**(2): 13–18.

Dawson J (1992) *Driving force for rural nursing practice*. Paper presented at the Australian Rural Health Conference, Infront, Outback.

Donnelly J (1993) *Registered Nurse Education and Training Needs*. South Eastern Health Region of NSW, New South Wales Health Rural Forum.

Dunne A (1995) Rural and remote nursing: what the textbooks don't tell you. In: D Hegney *et al.* (eds) *The Great Divide: Not Just a Mountain Range*. 4th Annual Conference of the Association for Australian Rural Nurses Inc., Toowoomba.

Dunning PL, Brown L, Phillips P and Ayers B (1994) Diabetes health care and education – the challenge of isolation. *The Australian Journal of Rural Health* **2**(3): 11–16.

Evans F (1994) The role of the registered nurse in the rural, but not remote, setting. *The Australian Journal of Rural Health* **2**(2): 15–18.

Fisher B (1993) *Setting the scene – a vision for district health*. Paper presented at the Rural Health Forum: New Networks – New Directions, Bowral.

Fuller D and Gartley B (1993) *Crossing the river and building bridges in a rural multicultural community*. Paper presented at Nursing the Country Conference of the Association for Australian Rural Nurses Inc., Warrnambool.

Hegney D (1995) Why do rural nurses continue to work in a role which is not legitimised? In: D Hegney *et al.* (eds) *The Great Divide: Not Just a Mountain Range.* 4th Annual Conference of the Association for Australian Rural Nurses Inc., Toowoomba.

Hegney D, Pearson A and McCarthy A (1998) *The Role and Function of the Rural Nurse in Australia.* Royal College of Nursing, Canberra.

Hodgson L (1992) Multiskilling: what does it mean for rural allied health? *The Australian Journal of Rural Health* **1**(1): 45–52.

Johnstone M (1992) Re-thinking the law, and challenging its traditional role in nursing's affairs: a strategy for professional reform. *Contemporary Nurse* **1**(1): 5–10.

Keyzer D (1994) Expanding the role of the nurse: nurse practitioners and case managers. *The Australian Journal of Rural Health* **2**(4): 5–11.

Keyzer D, Hall J, Mahnken J and Keyzer K (1995) *Gum Trees and Windmills: A Study in the Management of Time, Space and the Self-concepts of Community-based Nurses in One Rural Area of Victoria, Australia.* Deakin University, Warrnambool.

King J (1994) *Windmills, wisdom and wonderment: Can you find it all in Nursing?* Paper presented at the Windmills, Wisdom and Wonderment Conference of the Association for Australian Rural Nurses Inc., Roseworthy.

Kreger A (1991) *Report on the National Nursing Consultative Committee Project: enhancing the role of rural and remote area nurses.* Unpublished.

Lampshire P and Rolfe J (1991) *Great Expectations of the Community Health Nurse.* Health Department, Victoria.

Livingstone-Vail A (1994) Primary health care approach and quality outcomes in rural and remote settings. In: J Bailey, D du Plessis and D Lennox (eds) *2nd Biennial Australian Rural and Remote Health Scientific Conference.* Toowoomba.

McDonald H (1994) *Country practice: is it unique?* Paper presented at the Windmills, Wisdom and Wonderment Conference of the Association for Australian Rural Nurses Inc., Roseworthy.

NSW Health (1995) *Nurse Practitioner Project Stage 3.* NSW Health, Sydney.

Pearson A (1993) Expansion and extension of rural health workers' roles to increase access to health services in rural areas. In: K Malko (ed) *A Fair Go for Rural Health – Forward Together.* The University of New England, Armidale.

Spencer J (1994) *The education needs of undergraduate nurses in a rural nursing elective: curriculum evaluation and modification.* Paper presented at the Windmills, Wisdom and Wonderment Conference of the Association for Australian Rural Nurses Inc., Roseworthy.

Staunton PJ and Wyburn B (1989) *Nursing and the Law.* WB Sanders, Sydney.

Staunton P (1991) Nursing and the Law. In: ML Craig (ed) *A Fair Go for Rural Health.* Department of Health, Housing and Community Service, Canberra.

Vernon M (1994) *Multi-purpose services: what are they and how do they impact on rural nurses?* Paper presented at the Windmills, Wisdom and Wonderment Conference of the Association for Australian Rural Nurses Inc., Roseworthy.

CHAPTER EIGHT

Nurse practitioners in Australia

David White and Judi Brown

The evolution and recognition of the nurse practitioner role is one of the most important milestones in the history of nursing in Australia. Nurse practitioners are a viable alternative to other health professionals in terms of quality of care and cost effectiveness, and their introduction will provide a wider variety of consumer choice in healthcare.
(Australian Nurses Federation, 1999, cited in DHS, 1999b).

For some years in Australia, nurses and midwives in a variety of settings have provided services as nurse practitioner consultants and self-employed nurse practitioners (NPs). In many rural and most remote areas nurses already undertake the role, but to date no formal recognition has been afforded to these nurses in terms of the level of their skills. Whilst informal practice has been occurring for some time, formal recognition has become organised. The nurse practitioner movement in Australia has spanned the 1990s and is now growing steadily. It was launched in 1990, following a speech in New South Wales by the (then) Minister of Health. A working party was set up in 1992 to explore issues raised by the creation of this new role of independent nurse practitioner. The agreed definition of an NP was (NSW, 1993):

> *Nurse practitioners are registered nurses educated for advanced practice, the characteristics of which would be determined by the context in which they practice.*

A three-stage study was designed and pilot projects were initiated in three types of practice setting:

- remote areas
- general practice
- area/district health services.

In December 1995 NSW Health published the outcomes of the nurse practitioner trials. The report has 48 recommendations relating to issues such as recognition of the role of nurse practitioners, collaborative relationships between nurses and medical practitioners, accreditation education, the process for establishing nurse practitioner services, diagnostic imaging, diagnostic pathology, medications, referrals, funding, economic evaluation, professional indemnity, communication and publicity strategies (NSW, 1995). The report conclusively demonstrated that nurse practitioners can provide an efficient, cost-effective and highly skilled nursing service, whilst working collaboratively with the medical profession.

This latter finding (collaboration with medical colleagues) is an important one. If health workers are to meet the needs of the community they must work together more effectively. Expansion of the nurses' role is generally into the area of (previously perceived) 'medical' practice, most frequently because service needs to be given to under-served communities that are unable to attract doctors. Nurses extend and advance their skills to meet the range of practice that is required of them as the principal health worker in a community. Like in North America, however, the introduction of NPs has drawn a mixed response from the medical profession, who see their power base threatened.

Nurses have also felt constrained. Keyzer *et al.* (1995), in their study of practice and district nurses in rural Victoria, recommended that these nurses be given the education and training to work as NPs. They noted that the nurses were dependent on the medical officers' knowledge and control over their job content. They felt that medical dominance inhibited their role, and opportunities for independent practice. They went on to recommend a system of direct re-imbursement for nursing services which would overcome the *'wastage involved in unnecessary and indirect medical supervision'* of nurses.

New South Wales was the first state to have the title of nurse practitioner protected by legislation (NSW, 1998). This followed extensive collaborative work with key stakeholders who all had a vested interest in the area of practice to be offered by specially prepared NPs. A framework document was produced to guide implementation of NPs into the health service system. The framework document (NSW, 1998) outlined the policy and legislative changes that were to occur. Subsequently the Nurses' Amendment (Nurse Practitioners) Act, 1998 was passed by both houses of NSW parliament in September and October 1998.

The purpose of the Act is to:

- allow the Nurses Registration Board to authorise certain registered nurses to practice as nurse practitioners
- allow the Director-General of the DoH to approve guidelines related to the functions of NPs, and to allow such guidelines to make provision for the possession, use, supply and prescription of certain substances by NPs
- prevent an unauthorised person from using the title 'nurse practitioner' or otherwise holding himself or herself out to be a nurse practitioner.

It is stated that NPs will be specialist nurses with extensive knowledge, advanced skills and experience. They will work collaboratively with local medical practitioners and other members of the multi-disciplinary health team.

The document is far-sighted in that it enables, rather than disables the potential for development of innovative, community-responsive 'best practice'. The decision was made that it should be voluntary, rather than mandatory because:

- it does not confine nurses to areas where doctors do not wish to work
- accreditation is vested in the individual NP, not employee position.

Accreditation is granted, following successful application, by the Nurses Registration Board.

Offredy (1999) interviewed a policy adviser and discussed the reasons for the criteria chosen by the Board. He is reported as saying:

> We have not put restrictions or criteria so harsh that they would exclude people. The one issue that may be seen as exclusive is that within the legislation only nurses who are accredited as nurse practitioners will be able to call themselves by that title, so the title is restricted to people who have met the criteria for accreditation. In essence, this is not being inclusive, rather it is to establish a standard so that the public, employer or other health profession will know that if someone is a nurse practitioner, they . . . will have some idea of the level at which they (nurse practitioners) are working.

Offredy (1999) also explored the issue of advanced nursing practice in Australia. Particularly noteworthy here is the responsibility of the employer, as well as the practitioner. Commenting on the NSW (1998) framework document Offredy reports that:

The student will be required to demonstrate that he or she has met the criteria for accreditation as laid out in the framework document. The student will also need to provide evidence that he or she is practising at that level. The employer will also need to assess practice competence. Legally, the employer has an obligation to ensure that the right person is employed for the right job.

Although NSW has led the way in developing NPs in Australia, other states have also been active in developing this advanced nursing role. In Victoria, a task force has recommended and is awaiting funding for several pilot projects, and in Western Australia the working party is determining the appropriate knowledge and skills required by remote area nurses to provide safe, cost-effective care. A major project on nurse practitioners (NUPRAC – discussed below) has been undertaken in South Australia: the final report of the project was delivered to the Minister of Human Services in summer 1999. Two of the most significant outcomes are the clinical privileging and admitting privileging rights and processes that have been developed for nurse practitioners (South Australia is the first state to offer these in Australia).

The development of the nurse practitioner in South Australia

Although it is widely acknowledged in South Australia that some nurses/midwives already undertake a practitioner role, to date no formal recognition has been afforded to those nurses/midwives in terms of the level of their skills.

There is increasing evidence, however, that the further development and implementation of this role in a variety of settings will provide a significant addition to future healthcare models in this state and this development arises as a legitimate response to clients needs.

Role of the Department of Human Services

In November 1996, the Department of Human Services chose to take a leadership role in the development of a coordinated, collaborative approach to the recognition and development of the role of the nurse practitioner/midwife in advanced practice in South Australia.

The development of the strategic plan for this leadership process was strongly influenced by what was considered the most critical outcome from the NSW Nurse Practitioner Report, the *solid evidence* from the various trials regarding the nurse practitioner role and its place in the health system of the new millennium. It is from this evidence that opportunities to implement and further develop the model are being explored in South Australia.

In any promotion of the role and title of nurse practitioner, it has become increasingly important to emphasise that within the history of nursing and midwifery practice in South Australia there is strong and reliable evidence of the accepted status of the nurse practitioner role.

Current examples of advanced practice nurses in South Australia

Metropolitan

In the private health sector in South Australia there are currently 150 members of Nurses and Midwives in Private Practice, Australia (NAMIPPA) working in South Australia, with possibly two to three times more nurses working in private practice who do not belong to NAMIPPA.

Rural

Rural nurses and midwives in South Australia number 3031 (AIHW, 1996) or 18% of the state's registered nurses. This compares with about 3% for remote area nurses (RANs). Rural nurses and midwives work in a variety of clinical and community settings, ranging from a large regional hospital of 80–90 beds through to small community hospitals with fewer than ten beds.

There are no permanent resident medical officers in most rural hospitals and so rural nurses and midwives must provide a wide range of services, many of which are provided in the absence of a doctor in the first instance (for a fuller discussion of the work of rural nurses read Pearson *et al.* cited in Chapter Seven). Whilst it is acknowledged that not all rural nurses/midwives aspire to nurse practitioner status, some have been operating at this level for many years without legislative or professional sanction.

Remote

Remote area nurses work in consultation with doctors at a distance or with intermittent visiting doctors and specialists in primary health. At different times, the RAN works interdependently with doctors, other nurses, healthcare workers and ancillary personnel, such as X-ray technicians and pilots. Often alone or on frequent occasions, the RAN, with the most senior clinician available, makes judgements regarding whether to treat or refer presenting clients (McReynolds, 1998).

The South Australia Nurse Practitioner Project

Establishment of effective frameworks and facilitation of a coordinated approach is fundamental to all project initiatives and there is no doubt when the 'big picture' issues are tackled that frameworks, policies and definitions take on a new urgency and importance. The Department of Human Services (DHS) approach was to address these issues at the initial stage of the NUPRAC project development in order to minimise potential areas of difficulty or dispute and ensure that there was no fragmentation or isolation of roles. The initiation of the project included the establishment of an oversight committee – the Advisory Committee, and working groups – Reference Groups.

Advisory Committee

The Minister of Human Services established the Advisory Committee in June 1998 with the appointment of the Chairperson. Members of the Advisory Committee comprised representatives of significant stakeholders within the nursing and midwifery professions and broader healthcare services.

Reference Groups

Consultative input was maximised by the use of reference groups. These were established in October 1998 to examine the key outcomes identified as desirable by the Advisory Committee. Each reference group comprised members representative of a wide cross-section of key stakeholders. A key stakeholder was understood as a group who had specific expertise in the areas being explored. The following key areas were explored:

- education and preparation
- referrals
- prescribing and supply of medications
- diagnostic pathology and imaging
- communication and marketing.

Defining features of a nurse practitioner

Whilst at a national level it was deemed important that some consistency existed, it has become apparent during the progress of the project that there was a need to produce a collective view of the 'defining features' of a nurse practitioner in order to move on to identifying and resolving issues associated with the role and to avoid becoming preoccupied with definitions.

The defining features include the combined sub-roles of educator, mentor, provider, manager and researcher within the context of need, setting, education and autonomy. It is envisaged that the flexibility provided by the use of defining features will enable the profession to implement innovations in practice. Defining features are shown in Box 8.1

Box 8.1: Defining features of a nurse practitioner

- The combined role of educator, mentor, provider, manager and researcher.

Setting
- Relevant to the clinical context of practice in which the nurse practitioner wishes to be accredited.

Need
- Adds value and/or takes up or develops areas where existing work is not being done or where gaps in services exist.
- Consultation with other providers is necessary to ensure there is no duplication of services.

Educated, credentialled registered nurses who are experienced in the advanced practice role and:
- are experts in their special practice area
- are skilled in holistic care, case management and communication
- recognise the limits of their knowledge and practice

- meet the competency standards for advanced practice in their special practice area
- use evidence-based practice.

Autonomy

- Responsible and accountable for outcomes.
- Undergo accreditation through a formal process, including peer review.
- Take responsibility for continuing education.
- Work in collaboration with other healthcare providers.

Operational exemplars

To clarify and describe the types of services nurse practitioners/midwives might offer, exemplars have been used within the final report (DHS, 1999b). These exemplars serve to illustrate the role as well as the structures and support that nurse practitioners/midwives will need in order to undertake their roles successfully in the future.

In the *service-delivery* context, the role of the authorised nurse practitioner/midwife must be one in which they meet, either wholly or in part, a demonstrated service deficit or community need. Alternatively, or in addition, they may add value to the quality or range of services currently offered. The nurse practitioner/midwife adds value to existing services. To demonstrate this an operational exemplar for palliative care is shown in Box 8.2.

Box 8.2: An operational exemplar for palliative care

The **palliative care nurse practitioner** works in aged care facilities and her role incorporates consultancy, support, education and liaison for aged care facilities' staff, general practitioners, relatives and the residents who are dying.

The palliative care nurse practitioner provides a 24-hour, on-call service which includes the admission of clients, support for relatives and the provision of direct care to dying residents. To facilitate improvements in care and support of staff, the palliative care nurse practitioner also provides education for aged care facility staff. She also serves as a liaison between palliative care services and the aged care industry. She offers advice and support to general practitioners regarding treatment and management of clients in the terminal phase of life.

This exemplar illustrates how an authorised nurse practitioner who is able to offer services in palliative care can add value to existing services by enhancing the team approach through her specific expertise.

In the *relational* context, the nurse practitioner/midwife offers services that complement those already in existence. They inter-relate with relevant professional and non-professional colleagues in the course of their duties. There may be collaborative activities that they undertake with other health professionals.

Clinical and admitting privileges

The Department of Human Services is committed to primary health-care principles and support for nursing and midwifery interventions in a variety of settings. Emphasis is placed on providing particular support for those interventions that contribute to the fundamental role of the health system and where they directly enable the achievement of appropriate, safe and effective care outcomes.

The inability of nurses and midwives to be recognised via a clinical privileging process or to be able to admit and discharge patients for nursing care has been an area of professional concern. For nurse practitioners/midwives to contribute optimally to future healthcare models, a number of changes need to be made in the broader health arena. Clinical privileging is one of these areas.

In 1998–99 the Department of Human Services undertook extensive consultation with professional groups as part of a process to develop Admitting and Clinical Privileging guidelines (DHS, 1999a).

The guidelines, which are modelled on established medical guide-lines, were endorsed for distribution to health units in February 1999.

Outcomes of the nurse practitioner project

The final report of the NUPRAC project is in the process of presenta-tion to the Minister of Human Services through the Executive of the Department of Human Services. Its essence reflects the collaborative spirit in which the report was generated by the major stakeholders on the Advisory Committee. Implementation of the recommendations within the report, which includes legislation changes, establishment of an authorisation process by the Nurses Board of South Australia and development of education programmes, will provide significant structures and support systems for the development of the role of nurse practitioner in South Australia.

Comments from professional colleges and associations who assisted with the NUPRAC project

Royal College of Nursing, Australia (South Australia Chapter)

The Department of Human Services Nurse Practitioner Project is congruent with the Royal College of Nursing, Australia's Mission 'to benefit the health of the community through promotion and recognition of professional excellence in nursing'. The College believes the development of the nurse practitioner role is integral to the advancement of the nursing profession in Australia.

Australian Nurses' Federation

The evolution and recognition of the nurse practitioner role is one of the most important milestones in the history of nursing in Australia. Nurse practitioners are a viable alternative to other health professionals in terms of quality of care and cost-effectiveness, and their introduction will provide a wider variety of consumer choice in healthcare.

Australian Medical Association

Doctors have been working very closely with the nursing profession to develop the role of nurse practitioners in South Australia. The two professions are working at building on a modern complementary relationship.

The 'NuPrac Project' will achieve its outcome of seeing the medical and nursing professions complement each other in their work if it has a working understanding of the aims and directions intended for both professions. The reference groups have increased the understanding of how each profession works and their relationship with each other.

There are still some issues that have not been completely resolved, but I think that open communication and focusing on what is better for our community rather than protecting different patches and looking to usurp roles will allow the constructive relationship and exercise to continue.

Conclusions

The significance of nurse practitioners cannot be underestimated in the development of nursing for the 21st century. While the healthcare delivery system is undergoing massive changes there exist many opportunities. Nurse practitioners have much to offer and are much needed in many varied settings where demands for healthcare are greater than the availability of specific healthcare professionals to provide it. Their role will be challenged, but with standardised education, better public relations, and information justifying improved service quality and decreased costs, nurse practitioners will be well placed to meet the challenges and opportunities that lie ahead in the South Australian healthcare system.

References

AIHW (1996) *Nurse employee data*. Australian Institute of Health and Welfare.

DHS (1999a) *Guidelines for the Granting of Clinical Privileges and Admitting Privileges for Nurses and Midwives in Public Hospitals in South Australia.* Department of Human Services, Adelaide.

DHS (1999b) *Nurse practitioner project final report*. Department of Human Services, Adelaide. Unpublished.

Keyzer D, Hall J, Mahnken J and Keyzer K (1995) *Gum Trees and Windmills: A Study in the Management of Time, Space and the Self Concepts of Community-based Nurses in One Rural Area of Victoria, Australia.* Deakin University, Warrnambool.

McReynolds B (1998) *Remote area nurses working as nurse practitioners without the nurse practitioner training, education and recognition.* Poster presented at the 6th International Nurse Practitioner Conference, 5–8 Feb, Melbourne.

NSW (1993) *Nurse Practitioner Review Stage 2*. New South Wales Department of Health.

NSW (1995) *Nurse Practitioner Project Stage 3: Final Report of the Steering Committee*. New South Wales Department of Health.

NSW (1998) *The Framework for the Implementation of Nurse Practitioner Services in New South Wales*. New South Wales Department of Health.

Offredy M (1999) The nurse practitioner role in New South Wales: development and policy. *Nursing Standard* **14**(43): 38–41.

Nurse entrepreneurs for health

CHAPTER NINE

Making a difference

Marjorie Gott

> . . . *What we really need are social entrepreneurs for health.*
> (Everington, 1999)

Evidence presented in the preceding chapters of this book adds to a growing body of work that demonstrates nurses' ability to advance both nursing and health service practice to meet current healthcare needs. Conflicting requirements for healthcare in the 21st century, however, mean that nurses need to be aware of competing positions in the ongoing healthcare debate and to recognise the values that underpin them. They can then make more informed choices about both the way they wish to practice and their involvement in shaping policies to facilitate this.

The healthcare context

Competing ideologies exist in healthcare. On the one hand is the altruistic, socially inclusive approach of adherents to the WHO 'Health For All' (1978) philosophy, on the other is the view of health as a market commodity, to be bought (by those who can afford it). The moral dilemma implicit in these competing approaches is foreseen as problematic to the delivery of health services (WHO, 1997):

> *Health systems worldwide have failed to recognize the implications of the fundamental shift in the paradigm that has come to dominate economic and social development over the last decade. The paradigm can be paraphrased as 'the market approach'. It poses a number of fundamental*

challenges to the pursuit of health for all. These include advancement of the notion that health is merely a commodity, and as such has a price and can be traded off against other commodities . . . [what is needed is] a radical reorientation towards development of health systems whose goal is the improvement of the health status and well-being of entire populations, with priority to those in greatest need.

Reorientation of healthcare

In the early chapters of this book the worldwide health policy reorientation to primary healthcare was identified, as was the need for nurses and their colleagues to work differently with each other, and with the public. Calls for greater effectiveness and efficiency, increasing use of technology, demands for evidence-based practice and new professional roles in PHC mean that the clinical environment is changing rapidly and practitioners are becoming more selective in terms of skills and evidence (Dickson and Morrison, 1999):

Many primary healthcare teams approach the delivery of care in a multidisciplinary manner that attempts to use the best skills of all the team members in order to improve the quality of care provided to the patients. Future monitoring and research evaluation, related to the role of PHC nurses in evidence-based practice is required to maximise the impact of these nurses in relation to positive patient outcomes and good quality care.

Teamworking

More will be said about the need for evidence-based practice, for all health workers, in a later section; here the issue to emphasise is teamworking and respect for each others' skills. Several authors in previous chapters have commented on this welcome trend.

In her UK nurse practitioner study (Chapter Three), Chambers found, when she went back to visit her original research practices, that doctors believed that, following nurse call management, they were seeing far fewer acute minor illness episodes, that some surgeries were lighter, and they were managing more complex cases. Doctors believed that PHC workers were making greater use of each others' expertise.

This was also mentioned by Pearson *et al.* (Chapter Seven) who described the work of a rural general practice nurse following a new (nurse/doctor jointly designed and delivered) course of preparation for her role. Two nurses in the practice will soon have completed the course. There is now no perceived need in this practice to recruit additional general practitioners. It is reported that the current stable and high-functioning team have, through working with the community, identified needs and agreed on skilling staff within the team to meet these needs.

Good teamwork is necessary for innovation in PHC practice to develop and be sustained. Harrison and Neve (1996) looked for 'good practice' in, and carried out a review of, innovations in PHC. Criteria for successful innovation were:

- the use of an alliance or multi-agency team co-ordinated from a PHC setting
- the development of new primary care team members
- the deployment of existing team members with new skills (e.g. nurse practitioners).

They comment that the way that PHC has traditionally been delivered (doctors lead, others follow) needs to change.

Case studies of good practice in PHC have also been collected in the US, in a bid to reach out to and serve underserved and vulnerable groups in the population, (US DHHS, 1996). The *Models that Work* campaign promotes local PHC innovations that have been proved to work by stressing local control, best use of resources and results over process. The goal is to increase access to PHC, especially for the 43 million Americans without health insurance. An expert panel reviews nation-ally nominated PHC initiatives and selects, disseminates and builds on the good practice that is reported.

Good practice in PHC cannot develop in a climate of mistrust and protectionism in which professionals closely guard practice boundaries, thus stifle opportunities for innovation. Both Goodyear (Chapter Five) and Connors *et al.* (Chapter Six) raise this issue. They comment that problems of (doctor/nurse) competition for service delivery are almost nonexistent in rural/remote area care, but in more attractive areas, and when there is a fee-for-service payment involved to the physician, things are more problematic. Practitioners and policy makers now seem more aware of this, however, and there is a (fairly cautious) move towards collaboration, as opposed to competition (AMA, Chapter Eight):

> *There are still some issues that have not been completely*
> *resolved, but I think that open communication and focusing*
> *on what is better for our community rather than protecting*

different patches and looking to usurp roles will allow the
constructive relationship and exercise to continue.

In addition to problems caused by 'turf wars', there are also problems
related to changing the system. The healthcare system is huge, bureaucratic and full of vested interests working to maintain the (non-
threatening) status quo. The difficulties of building innovative practice
in a bureaucratic system have been commented on by Everington
(1999):

> *The traditional local authority is top-down, heavily bureau-*
> *cratic and slow. It's difficult to work with them and get them*
> *to change services. Real change is people driven and starts at*
> *the margins and grows upwards. What we really need are*
> *social entrepreneurs for health.*

Managing care: use of common protocols

Interdisciplinary care recognises and utilises the different skills of team
members, but the margins of care and responsibility are blurred and
shared. Leaders are more likely to work jointly and collaboratively, to
commonly agreed protocols of good practice. Depending upon the issue
and the context, protocols are as likely to be devised by nurses as by
doctors or other team workers.

The use of common, jointly (nurse/doctor) developed protocols to
manage care incidents seems critical to success. Chambers found that,
using protocols and guidelines, it was easier to run the organisation
with the key participants all working in the same way. Protocols were
also mentioned by Bamford in her study of a NLMIU (Chapter Four).
The unit had protocols for practice, the majority of which were the
result of joint development between medical and nursing staff. Jointly
developing these allowed ownership of practice decisions to build, thus
making the change in practice more stable. Communications between
nurses and doctors were also improved. Bamford raises an important
issue to do with standards, however, when she comments on the fact
that some protocols in the unit surveyed were not adopted from
national guidelines, and thus threatened standards of care. She identifies a need to develop common standards and protocols for this area of
care and sees evidence-based practice as the cornerstone for these
developments.

Working together on a problem builds ownership of the solutions
arrived at. Several contributors to this book have emphasised this; the
authors of Chapter Eight (describing the South Australia Nurse Practi-

tioner Project) built ownership in as part of their development strategy by early involvement of all key stakeholders (those with a vested interest in the outcome of the project).

Serving the community: needs driven service development

Many examples of nurses seeking out and meeting the needs of their various communities have been provided in this book. Some are led by practice, others by education (UK educator, Chapter Two):

> . . . the student thought that they were getting second-rate care and so she put the case to managers and that's been pursued by the health trust to develop either a leg ulcer clinic in that area, or look at training staff to give the care there.

The most significant development, across countries, has been that of the nurse practitioner role. Nurse practitioners offer the public an alternative (non-doctor) first point of contact into the health system. As Chambers outlines (Chapter Three) nurse practitioners have the authority to examine, diagnose and treat, following protocols agreed with the doctors, where appropriate, as well as utilising a holistic model of care, with a health advice and promotion focus.

The development of the nurse practitioner role is making a significant contribution to healthcare. It has not been an easy evolution, however; there has been hostile resistance to the role from outside and within the profession (*see* Chapter One). Except in the US (where NP growth and practice is limited by the expansion of private healthcare organisations), the NP role is set to expand. The story of the development of the NP in the US, however, is one that should be closely examined. There are lessons here that should be instructive for other countries as they seek to develop this advanced practice nursing role. Particular attention should be paid to the way in which professional organisation, appropriate education, setting of standards and credentialling have been achieved. Those seeking a template for development of the role, should also look to Chapter Eight, in which thorough, insightful, and inclusive development processes are outlined.

Bamford (Chapter Four) and Pearson *et al.* (Chapter Seven) describe the success of the extended role of the nurse in meeting the needs of communities. Bamford reports on the extended clinical practice nurse working as the first point of contact in a community-based A&E service and provides evidence to support the assertion that this is an area of practice that is seen as successful and growing. This is because it is cost-effective, well liked by patients and a more appropriate form of (PHC) service delivery than high-cost, doctor-led A&E care. The nurse-led minor injuries (NLMI) service is a form of provision that operates on the principles of PHC (first point of contact for treatment/referral), but is delivered in a secondary care institution (community hospital). Small (community) hospitals are under threat of closure as specialist services increasingly become grouped into large city 'super' hospitals (centres of excellence in disease management). As these changes occur, health policy makers and managers are going to need to ensure that innovative forms of community-based service delivery are protected. If they do not (expensive) misuse of services will occur. Tanaka *et al.* (1994), for example refer to inappropriate ambulance use by non-emergency patients in Japan:

> *The insufficient development of primary healthcare resources and systems increased the inappropriate use of high-cost emergency ambulance services by the elderly living in urban areas . . . Health systems therefore need to be re-orientated so as to enhance accessibility to primary health-care services.*

Relocation and concentration of some health services may also threaten accessibility to care. Some communities, however, are already chronically underserved or neglected. Pearson *et al.* (Chapter Seven) cite rural nurses as serving the community by providing a full range of nursing and health services, which no other professionals would provide:

> *with the current reluctance of medical practitioners to work in small rural areas and the inability of health services to employ a range of allied health professionals (due to the cost), if nurses did not 'fill the gap', the service would not be provided. Therefore, extended practice roles are essential to the provision of health services in rural areas.*

Goodyear (Chapter Five) also speaks of nurses delivering an extended range of services to previously underserved (poor) rural communities in the southern US. In the face of major obstacles one family nurse practitioner (with extended and advanced skills) set up her own practice. It was highly successful. Six years down the road, however, she ran into the managed care juggernaut. Health policy changes, caused by the growth of HMOs, meant wholesale registration of residents of states into managed care programmes. The FNP could no longer practice. Goodyear reports:

At the turn of the 21st century, nine years after the practice was started, this issue remains unresolved. The practice was closed after six years of active successful service to a community of over 500 families. These families have had to be placed with other practices in the community or in the surrounding community. The economists would not consider this endeavour a success, the physicians would indicate the same. However, the nurse practitioner, colleagues, students and patients see positive outcomes. The demonstration was of a nurse practitioner, initiating and implementing a private practice based on a nursing model, providing unparalleled service for a period of six years.

Patient satisfaction with services

In the UK, the US and Australia, patients and clients are satisfied with nurse-run services. Chambers (Chapter Three) cites those respondents who consulted the nurse practitioner as giving statistically significant higher satisfaction scores for the nurse in comparison with the doctor, using the four parameters of listening, explaining, information and time. She provides other research on patient satisfaction ratings for nurse practitioners to corroborate this finding. There was also evidence that patients particularly liked the speedy access to a health professional that the NP service provides.

According to Bamford (Chapter Four) the public understand, accept and value a nurse-led minor injuries service. Services are able to offer a quick response to individuals, and to provide reassurance. She goes on to report that there does not seem to be an issue in most people's minds about whether they are seen by a doctor or a nurse. They just want to be seen by someone and have their problem dealt with. They trusted the nurse to refer them to a doctor if it was thought necessary.

This finding is in line with that of Everington (1999) who describes the success of a new emergency service based in a deprived inner-London area. A local co-operative of (75) GPs work on a voluntary basis to support A&E staff at the local hospital to provide 24-hour PHC and emergency services. According to Everington, 80% of healthcare happens in PHC. The co-operative offers phone advice, services to 'walk ins' and emergency care. It is successful and heavily used. The plan is to incorporate nurse led services, such as minor injuries (Everington, 1999):

What people want is an immediate response to their fears; a doctor on the phone gives that straight away.

Nurses working in rural areas in both the US and Australia also offer this type of response, advice and care service (Chapters Five and Seven).

Cost-effectiveness

Universally, educated nurses working in an extended or advanced practice role are cost-effective healthcare providers. They would be even more cost-effective if their practice was not limited by law (lack of sufficient prescribing and of admitting privileges in the UK) or unchecked market forces (growth of Managed Health Care Organisations in the US). Goodyear (Chapter Five) reports a special issue of the *Yale Journal on Regulation* addressing the under-utilisation of nurse practitioners as a means of resolving the spiralling costs of healthcare. Also highlighted is restraint in achieving the full potential of NPs, due partly to the regulating agencies across the nation.

Chambers (UK) and Goodyear (US) in Chapters Three and Five, show that, within a range of PHC practice, nurse practitioners are as effective as, and cheaper than doctors. For Australia, White and Brown (Chapter Eight) cite the New South Wales report (1995):

> *The report conclusively demonstrated that nurse practitioners can provide an efficient cost effective and highly skilled nursing service, whilst working collaboratively with the medical profession.*

The finding is also true for those working in an extended (as opposed to advanced) role. Pearson *et al.* report rural nurses as cost-effective (Chapter Seven) and Bamford (Chapter Four) reports the same for the nurse-led minor injuries service:

> *Nearly 60% of patients were seen by, diagnosed, treated and discharged by the nurses working in the department. Comparing the nurse run service and the medical-run large hospital A&E service, the same outcome occurred in 165 (59%) instances. That is the same outcome if the person was cared for in the NLMI unit or the high technology (medically managed) A&E department. This leads to the conclusion that many minor illness and injuries can be dealt with by experienced and well-prepared nurses.*

She goes on to say:

(incidence) . . . *would probably have been higher but poor records made it difficult to match cases.*

In addition to cost savings through better management practices, several studies show that nurses with more education deliver more cost-effective care (Buchan, 1994).

Nursing standards, competence and evidence-based practice

This was an issue of concern for authors of preceding chapters. Talking about UK NPs, Chambers (Chapter Three) says:

> *There is no national standard, therefore, it is difficult for employers and colleagues to know what NPs have to offer. A local solution to the training problem might be a combination of the externally provided and validated course, such as the one now franchised by the Royal College of Nursing, with practice-based training with a GP mentor, in order for the doctors in the practice to develop confidence in sharing clinical decision making with a non-medical colleague.*

Talking of the nurse-led minor injuries service, Bamford (Chapter Four) cites standards as problematic because there is no formal recognition of the role, thus a lack of 'benchmarking' and specific educational preparation. She also comments on the lack of continuing education opportunities, partly caused by lack of managerial guidance, provision and support.

Maintenance of standards and lack of continuing education opportunities are also raised by Pearson *et al.* (Chapter Seven), who identify the 'Catch 22' situation in which Australian rural nurses practice:

> *First, it is acknowledged that rural nurses are experiencing difficulty in accessing continuing professional education, which is necessary to ensure that they are competent and confident in their practice. One would expect, therefore, that those who have not been able to access current information are not working to an accepted standard. Second, there is no agreed standard for rural nursing practice. The question remains: what is this standard and by what scope of practice criteria is it judged?*

Like Bamford, these authors also cite employer responsibility as a factor in variability of standards of service:

> *Employers continue to employ nurses in these extended practice roles with full knowledge that the majority of them have been ill-prepared for their role. . . . [there is] concern over the 'double standard' which expects the practitioner to practise beyond their level of preparation with nil (or limited) professional support, no legislative support nor industrial support and limited opportunities for professional development.*

The situation needs to be addressed urgently. There are some signs that it now is, but the spread of best (evidence-based) practice may be slow to reach some areas. This will be due to the prevailing attitudes and support practices of managers, as much as to geography.

Accessing resources will improve, however. Owing to the relatively accessible, low-cost (phone line, local rates) technological resources of the Internet, finding out about good nursing practice is becoming easier. Collaboration is also increasing as networks and websites of good practice in nursing care develop and expand. Evers (1997) calls for the initiation of permanent data collections of nursing data on a European scale and cites existing European projects (Telenursing, WISECARE) as the way forward in collaborative data collection and dissemination. A number of university-based organisations around the world provide information on collections of resources. Useful for NPs, for example, is the Internet Resources for Nurse Practitioners Guide, provided on-line by the University of San Francisco (data at nursing@ccmail.ucsf.edu).

The Centre for Evidence-Based Nursing at the University of York (UK), like the Joanna Briggs Institute (Adelaide, Australia) is an international resource of peer-reviewed, evidence-based nursing practice (http://www.joannabriggs.edu.au), (www.york.ac.uk/depts/hstd/centres/evidence/ev-intro.htm).

In addition to more opportunities for adoption of evidence-based best practice, the requirement for clinical audit, in which peers review colleagues' practice, should also lead to general improvement in standards of care.

In the UK, standards of quality care are now set and monitored nationally, and delivered locally by a package of measures known as clinical governance. The goal is to safeguard standards of care and enhance quality. The four main components are (Roland *et al.*, 1999):

- structures to promote clear lines of responsibility and accountability
- quality improvement programmes

- risk management
- support frameworks to identify and improve poor performance.

It is worth commenting here that however good the monitoring systems devised (whatever country), they will be worthless unless clear job-related competencies are identified, and appropriate education and regular continuing education opportunities are provided. This is particularly urgent for those nurses who are vulnerable (for example, working in non-traditional ways/settings). Otherwise, the danger is that monitoring systems will become a tool to beat nurses with (victim blaming of 'bad' practitioners), rather than a liberating force for the profession.

Competencies for the extended/advanced nursing role should be decided by the requirements of the population to be served, in consultation and collaboration with other healthcare providers (if these exist). Regarding the US, Clements (1997) talks of how standards and protocols have been developed in a public health nursing service to meet the needs of the underserved and uninsured population. Traditionally, public health services had delivered care to whole communities. The growth of private care organisations, however, has fragmented provision and left some people potentially uncared for. Paradoxically the public health service that has developed, rather than becoming just a safety net for 'second rate' citizens, is a truly consumer needs driven health programme. Clements describes a programme in which services are delivered according to established standards of care and outcomes are formally measured by Peer Review and Quality Assurance Committees. Written policies and objectives in turn provide medical and nursing directives for specific health programmes. She cites, as an example, protocols for the pregnancy testing programme, which include agreed interventions for positive and negative results.

Increasingly, evidence-based practice will be related to the development of Centres of Excellence. In the UK, a National Institute for Clinical Excellence has been established (1999), to issue guidance on best practice to achieve clinical and cost-effectiveness. Some existing centres are nurse initiated. These are mostly in metropolitan areas, but Leipert and Retter (1998) report on a community nurse partnership with women in remote parts of Canada and the setting up of Centres of Excellence to support best practice:

> *The five Centres for Excellence for Women's Health will help facilitate research activities, knowledge collection and dissemination, and the development of policies that will enhance women's health and community health nursing practice in geographically isolated settings.*

Reorientation of professional education

The need for a more relevant education for their role has been identified by nurses working in minor injuries units (Chapter Four), rural nursing (Chapter Seven) and UK NPs in primary healthcare (Chapter Three). Bamford (Chapter Four) argues that lack of adequate education threatens standards of care and militates against teamworking. She sees this as compounding professional prejudices about who can provide what type of care to patients.

Goodyear (Chapter Five), speaking of early development of the NP role in the US, comments that:

> *A variety of programs, different program lengths and no consistent curriculum threatened the credibility of the nurse practitioner.*

She goes on to report that the requirement of all nurse practitioners to be prepared at a recognised (Master's) level, in an accredited programme, has helped make knowledge uniform and testable. Standard-setting and benchmarking can thus occur. In the US, development of curricular guidelines by the NONPF was seen as instrumental in guiding programmes to prepare nurse practitioners at a level of competence in graduate education. Collaborative work occurred between accrediting bodies, faculties and governmental agencies with the aim of achieving this goal. Australia is also following this path, but the UK is lagging seriously behind. The regulatory body (UKCC) needs to broaden its gaze, speed up its decision making and benefit from the successful developments in America (described in Chapter Five) and Australia (Chapter Eight).

Health policy leaders and experts have delivered a 'call for action' to health professions schools to develop greater and improved community competencies among their students (in the US the Pew Health Professions Commission, 1995, in the UK the Department of Health *Strategy for Nursing* 1999, in Australia the New South Wales and South Australia governments: *see* Chapter Eight).

CCPH (*see* Chapter Six) stands as a case study of good practice in providing leadership at a national level in reorientation of health professional education. Students involved in service–learning are expected to not only provide direct community service but also to learn about the context in which the service is provided, the connection between the service and their academic coursework, and their roles as citizens. Service–learning efforts supported by the institution influenced the breakdown of the 'ivory tower' and inaccessible campus image. Establishing an Office of Community Programs at the university provided a link between the community and the institution. Before the establishment of this office, the community would have been less likely to view the university as a (local) community resource.

In addition to sensitivity and flexibility, a commitment to excellence and to lifelong learning is required by health professionals (Ashton 1998). Urging change (multi-disciplinary learning) in medical education, Stuart (1999) says:

> [there are] . . . *implications for changes in our most fundamental concepts of medical education and practice, in society's health awareness and expectations, in the roles and responsibilities of individual citizens, in the commitment and accountability of all levels of health professionals.*

This is particularly true of the US. A number of innovations are associated with university professional education centres. UCLA School of Nursing, for example, provides the Rescue Mission Centre in downtown Los Angeles where nurse practitioners (and trainees) give primary and preventive care and health education to multi-ethnic, homeless families. Now in its second decade, this initiative provides culturally relevant assessment and management of primary health problems, such as violence and abuse. It is also a gateway to other illness, health and welfare services. The service is context sensitive and is 'bottom up', so conditions for sustained change, over the longer term, are met.

Limits to progress

The healthcare market

In spite of well-developed education support systems, additional federal government funding to increase their number, and a high degree of political awareness about what was happening in the healthcare context, American NPs have been frustrated in their efforts to practice. NPs are faring better in Australia: legislation for autonomous advanced nursing practice is now in place, but the position is less good in the UK, where NPs have the opportunity to practice, but no protection through legislation or specific educational preparation.

Both the UK and Australia are experiencing expansion of the private sector into the healthcare 'market'; expansion of the nursing role may therefore be threatened. Of course educated advanced practice nurses are good value for money, and this might be recognised and exploited by the private healthcare industry, but the lesson provided by the US case studies (Chapter Five), in which NPs were squeezed out of service delivery, is a chilling one, and one which nurses practising in other 'advanced' societies worldwide should note. In doing so they might also reflect on the way these US NPs are fighting back. They are politically astute and entrepreneurial, and proactive with regard to managing change in a chaotic healthcare context.

The law

Some nurses are hindered by lack of nurse prescribing and admitting and referral rights. Nurses running minor injuries units in the UK describe being forced to call for GP advice because the patients that they were dealing with fell into areas of treatment which at that time could not be dealt with fully by nurses, because of policy or statutory limitations. These limitations include prescribing authority and/or referral authority to request further investigations within the NHS (Chapter Four).

With regard to rural general practice nurses (Australia), Pearson *et al.* (Chapter Seven) report a high degree of autonomy on the part of these practitioners, but indicate that this operates on a tenuous, *ad hoc,* 'grace and favour' basis, rather than being legally proscribed. These authors also believe that rural nurses are limited by the lack of prescribing rights.

In the US, Goodyear (Chapter Five) describes nurses who, although lacking formal education in business and entrepreneurial skills, demonstrate a high level of political awareness and flexibility. She believes that, in many instances, this has paid off for them; however, in some instances they remain limited by external factors, such as the expansion of the healthcare market, protectionist professional practices and restrictive legislation.

Against this backdrop the decision by the South Australian government (*see* Chapter Eight) to grant NPs clinical, admitting and prescribing privileges is to be welcomed. Other Australian states and other countries should watch progress here, and learn from it.

Institutional opposition

Community–campus partnerships for health have been cited as an example of good practice in reorientating the education of health professions (Chapter Six). Nurse educators working in educational institutions may recognise the need for this type of innovatory education, but, due to poor institutional leadership, be powerless to implement change. One US educator (*see* Chapter Two) designed a new, community needs-led course but it was not approved; she recalls feeling like an alien when she proposed it:

> . . . *This kind of multi-sectoral working is a very low priority, no matter what they say. They just give it lip service.*

Interestingly, multi-sectoral working is listed as a goal in the five-year plan of the institution. The School of Nursing leadership is failing here; just such a course is required to serve this community's unique needs (there is a regular influx of refugees across a national border line). It is worth exploring what was proposed by the educator.

As part of the Advanced Community Nursing Practicum a multi-disciplinary course was proposed. The course objectives were that students be able to:

* assess physical and psychosocial health needs of newly arriving refugee families
* develop, through community asset mapping, a resource manual specific to the selected population's community
* provide culturally appropriate healthcare to a refugee population group
* apply public health concepts to healthcare across clinical settings (includes referrals and follow-up for various services needed by newly arriving refugees)
* develop proficiency in working in a multidisciplinary team, with each member providing an aspect of care for which he or she is responsible, and with the shared goal of assisting the population group to achieve their optimum health
* participate in a variety of reflective activities which may include journalling, tape-recordings, discussion groups, etc.
* recognise the civic and social responsibilities of nurses as community leaders/advocates.

It is difficult to see how such a contextually sensitive and academically sound proposal would be rejected by faculty, but it was. This educator now gets peer support and professional enrichment from her activities outside the institution.

Regulating and validating bodies

If the profession of nursing is to progress and advance, practitioners must work to a recognised, recordable standard. Lack of registration also means lack of a career pathway. This in turn leads to recruitment and retention problems (WHO, 1996):

> *Deployment of nurses with higher education in nursing practice requires a career structure for nurses within the healthcare system. Without such a career structure (which must include conditions for autonomy in practice and adequate renumeration) the potential contribution of well-educated nurses as leaders in the development of nursing practice and improved healthcare services may be lost.*

Lack of agreement on the scope and level of practice for recordable qualification on the professional register affecting UK NPs has been commented on earlier. This problem has been recognised by the nursing statutory body for a number of years, but not acted on. Working groups continue to deliberate on the development of a revised regulatory framework for post-registration clinical practice, meanwhile nurses get on with expanding their practice to meet changes and challenges. Walsh (1999) recognises the frustration that these nurses are feeling:

> *NPs are part of a grassroots movement, growing organically from the bottom up, to meet healthcare needs . . . they are ordinary nurses frustrated at the limitations imposed on them. They can see the benefits to patients of taking further education and being allowed to practice more autonomously.*

The statutory body, the UKCC, has spent years deliberating about level of practice. Although NPs are now recognised as advanced level (therefore autonomous) practitioners in Australia and the US, the current thinking at UKCC is that the level for UK NPs will be set below the 'Higher Level', at specialist practitioner level (personal communication, August 1999). This will cause further confusion in the profession in the UK, not least because the government has stolen a march on nursing leadership with the publication of the *Strategy for Nursing* document (DoH, 1999b) which clearly sets out four levels of practice:

- a basic grade of healthcare assistant
- a main grade of qualified nurse
- a further grade with advanced qualifications
- a 'supernurse' grade of consultant practitioner.

In the UK, nursing leadership hovers on the threshold, afraid to enter the bigger debate about what kind of healthcare we need and how we can best deliver it. Politicians have made up their minds. They can see the worth of nurse-led services, and are providing opportunities to extend them (DoH, 1999a). So can innovative practitioners, who are familiar with grassroots needs, and have evolved new practices to meet them. Leaders of the profession stand in their way.

Lack of autonomy

Autonomy is vital if nurses working in advanced and extended practice are to achieve their potential and make a real difference to healthcare. Just as suffragettes won political enfranchisement early in the 20th century, nurses need to win practice enfranchisement early in the 21st. Nurses need the power to practice. Powerful practice will increase the visibility of nursing and alter perceptions of the difference nursing can make. Smart nurses know this; as the example below illustrates.

As previously indicated, NPs are good value for money, and will practice with all client populations. This can work to their advantage. Lardner (1998) describes a New York City initiative in which (Medicare and other) clients' health needs are met exclusively by a group of nurse practitioners who diagnose, treat, prescribe, refer and bill in the same way as doctors. Nurses get the same fee for service rates as doctors. The service originated from the University of Columbia School of Nursing programme which, in 1993 was asked to help in providing health services to two poor upper Manhattan neighbourhoods. The Dean of Nursing, Mary Mundinger recognised the politics involved in the invitation and asked for greater nurse practitioner scope to make the service more effective. The service has now spread to some affluent neighbourhoods. The public like nurse-run practices and are welcoming them as a new branch of primary health care. Lardner cites other studies which show that the care NPs provide is at least equal to that of physicians, and that nurses are better at communication and patient education.

The curriculum

A major concern for many nurses, discussed in the preceding chapters, is that there is no agreed or recognised form of preparation for their expanded role. They, and the public, need protection by agreement on, and provision of appropriate curricula. Nurses need to develop the skills to make a difference to healthcare services. Currently, leadership, business and management of change skills are under-represented, or absent in existing post-registration curricula. This issue will be explored in Chapter Ten.

Nurses also need to be prepared for involvement in policy making (Australian lecturer):

> . . . if they're going to be effective healthcare practitioners, which we're aiming for them to be, if they don't understand the policy process and if they don't understand its political way and its contested nature then they're not going to be effective.

The way education is delivered also needs to change. Uniprofessional education of health professionals should be the exception, rather than the norm. If health professionals are required to work together in service-delivery teams they need to problem solve together as students. Nurse educators have made some attempts to involve medical students in shared education, but met with very poor attendance from them. Medical educators need to pay heed. PHC is not a one-man (woman) band. Respect and proper use of each others skills means understanding and co-developing them.

Conclusions: the need to showcase nursing skills

Working in a range of settings, from inner-city areas to remote communities, nurses have shown that they can make a difference to healthcare. Across a range of health services they deliver care that is at least equal to that provided by other health workers (principally doctors), and, in some cases, better. They are flexible, multi-skilled, cost-effective, well-accepted by communities and are keen to develop new skills and advance their education. They are worthy of far more attention and investment than they have previously experienced.

There is a need for new autonomous clinical roles and career structures for senior clinical nurses; these roles need to be developed in partnership with other health professionals and be driven by clearly identified health and illness care demands generated by local communities. Professional education will need to change. It will need to be more responsive to both the needs of students and the needs of communities. In addition, service, management and education need to work together more effectively.

All nurses would benefit from better political and marketing skills. In developing these skills nurses need to follow through some challenging issues which they have previously sidelined, such as the scope and value of advanced clinical skills and their relationship with medicine and public health work.

References

Ashton J (1998) Health for all: from myth to reality. *Changing Medical Education and Medical Practice*. World Health Organisation, Geneva.

Buchan (1994) *Further Flexing? NHS trusts and changing working patterns in NHS nursing*. Royal College of Nursing, London.

Clements BJ (1997) Public health nursing services. *Witchita Falls Medicine* **12**(3): 7–10.

DoH (1999a) *Making a Difference. Strengthening the nursing, midwifery and health visiting contribution to health and healthcare*. Department of Health, London.

DoH (1999b) *Strategy for Nursing*. Department of Health, London.

Dickson R and Morrison C (1999) Nursing and evidence-based practice: a world away from evidence-based health. In: M Gabbay (ed) *The Evidence-Based Primary Care Handbook*. Royal Society of Medicine, London.

Everington S (1999) Primary care. *Socialist Health Association Conference* July 26. London

Evers GCM (1997) The future role of nursing and nurses in the European Union. *European Nurse* **2**(3): 171–9.

Harrison L and Neve H (1996) *A Review of Innovations in Primary Health Care*. The Policy Press, Bristol, UK.

Lardner J (1998) For nurses, a barrier broken. *US News & World Report* **July 27**: 58–61.

Leipert B and Reutter L (1998) Women's health and nursing practice in Canada. *Health Care for Women International* **19**(6): 575–88.

Roland M, Holden J and Campbell S (1999) *Quality Assessment for General Practice: Supporting Clinical Governance in Primary Care Groups*.

National Primary Care Research and Development Centre, University of Manchester.

Stuart K (1999) The National Health Service: doctors and society beyond 2000. *Journal of the Royal Society of Medicine* **92**: 142–5.

Tanaka A, Takehito T and Nakamura K (1994) Inappropriate use of emergency ambulance services and the implications for primary healthcare in Japan. *Health Promotion International* **9**(4): 259–68.

US Department of Health and Human Services (1996) *Models That Work, Compendium of Innovative Primary Health Care Programs for Under-served and Vulnerable Populations.* Bureau of Primary Health Care, Washington.

Walsh M (1999) Nurses and nurse practitioners part 2: perspectives on care. *Nursing Standard OnLine: Research* 1–10.

WHO (1978, and subsequent) *Alma Ata Declaration* (on Health For All). WHO Regional Office for Europe, Copenhagen.

WHO (1996) *Nursing Practice. Report of a WHO Expert Committee.* Technical Report No 860. World Health Organisation, Geneva.

WHO (1997) *Primary Healthcare Systems and Services for the 21st Century. Statement of the Seventh Consultative Committee on Organisation of Health Systems Based on Primary Health Care.* World Health Organisation, Geneva.

CHAPTER TEN

Nursing practice, policy and change: the future

Marjorie Gott

> *Nurses, midwives and health visitors are often constrained by structures that limit development and innovation.* (Blair, 1999)

At the beginning of this book it was stated that, in spite of being the largest professional group within the health services, nursing, as a profession, is anxious and insecure about its future. It shouldn't be. As the authors of the previous chapters have shown, given the opportunity, nurses can effectively and efficiently advance service delivery to meet a broad spectrum of health and illness care need. Given the right kind of education, management and legislative support they could be a significant force in meeting healthcare demands in this new century (Adebadjo, 1998).

The healthcare context

The 1990s have seen increasing policy commitment to (within budget) reorientation of healthcare towards care in the community. Switching efforts and resources from secondary (hospital) to primary (community-based) care is now the main policy direction of all western governments. Governments need to recognise that nurses are uniquely placed and prepared to help them in their efforts; nurses already have a broader holistic mind set than other PHC workers, they are also willing to accept change in the way they practice. Nurses can influence policy by showcasing good practice that works, and can be sustained over time.

Invariably this will be community responsive bottom-up development, rather than ('big business'/central government) top-down change.

Buxton *et al.* (reported in Salvage, 1999) see the growth of (community) nurses use of evidence-based practice in their day-to-day work as evidence of their willingness to embrace change:

> *While some managerial respondents referred to nurses as being generally traditional and resistant to change, practitioners indicated high levels of commitment to the principle of research-based practice.*

These nurses were very clear about how they could be helped to develop better practice:

> *Time to think about it and reduced workloads. Time to discuss it with somebody knowledgeable. Support in doing it. Reward for having done it.*

The principal reward that nurses want is the time, support and power to nurse as they feel they should. They also want the space and autonomy that role extension and flexibility can provide. Changes in PHC service delivery are starting to allow for this.

The inter-professional rivalries and 'turf wars' that characterised 20th century healthcare were in no one's long-term interest; and certainly not the patients that the system is meant to serve. The current world-wide reorientation of healthcare, with its emphasis on collaborative development of good practice demands both that health professionals work together more effectively, and that governments more rigorously address the value they are getting for the healthcare dollar, and who best can deliver it. Traditional views, roles and practices will change as these issues are addressed. According to Seifer (1997):

> *In the future, the most valued students entering the healthcare workforce will be those who are prepared to know more things in broad ways, and to transfer this knowledge in more collaborative teams in community-based settings.*

New clinical skills and new managerial skills are needed. There continues to be resistance to the expansion of those clinical skills required for the type of autonomous practice advocated throughout this book. Strong resistance is evident amongst nurses themselves. This is because some nurses see expansion of nurses technical skills as the practice of medicine, not nursing.

Talking about the development of the role of the nurse practitioner in the US Goodyear (Chapter Five), reports that:

> *A controversy between nurse educators preparing nurse practitioners and educators of traditional nurses was the perception that the expanded scope of practice was not nursing. The new curriculum content was viewed as medicine . . . and was met with scepticism, outrage and doubt.*

She goes on to comment that the reaction was as much a (to be expected) resistance to change, than the nature of the change itself. Nurses, especially those working in large institutions, like educators and service managers, are generally resistant to change; pressure comes upwards from practitioners, as they seek to respond to shifting social forces. Building acceptance of, and preparation for change into institutions is discussed in more detail in a following section: here the accompanying issue is one of responding to changed service needs.

The 'what is (and is not) nursing' debate is an incestuous one that serves the profession ill; if we don't make our minds up, others (governments, the market) will. The education issues of professional versus technical nursing continue to be intensely debated by the profession's leaders, but, after half a century, remain unresolved. In the meantime, nursing practice has been tailored by economic forces and public policy. The nursing profession itself, however, and some of the statutory bodies that govern education and training, seem unaware that the world is changing but persist in professional protectionism that separates nurse from nurse and hinders both the profession of nursing and innovation in service delivery.

Healthcare in the future will be more fluid and flexible: substitution of the skills of various professional workers will allow for redistribution of tasks. Substitution was part of the 'Heathrow Debate' on the future of nursing (1994). It is seen as:

> *the continual regrouping of resources across and within care settings, to exploit the best and least costly solutions in the face of changing needs and demands.*

Education and practice: serving the community

Increasingly, there will be collaboration rather than competition in PHC practice and preparation for practice (Hine, 1999). The (UK) Royal College of Nursing undertook a futures project in which: *'ordinary nurses were encouraged to think about the future.'* It reported in 1998. Education for nursing was still seen as too limiting by many participants. One said:

> *In a world where we are all supposed to be working across boundaries in the interests of patients, we need to be taught across them as well.*

The shared goal of community responsiveness is driving both nursing and medical post-basic education. Reporting on a collaborative venture between education and service De Maeseneer and Derese (1998) describe the 'community curriculum' provided for medical students at the University of Washington:

> *The rural/underserved opportunity program places medical students in practitioners' offices in order to realize the three major objectives:*
>
> - *to expose students to community medicine*
> - *to encourage students to develop positive attitudes towards rural and undeserved community medicine*
> - *to provide students with opportunities to learn how the local healthcare systems function.*

Doctors and nurses are also collaborating on education for new nursing roles. In the UK and US many nurse practitioner programmes began by nurses working side-by-side with supportive physician colleagues determining the course content intending nurse practitioners would need to provide service in an primary health/community care setting. In Australia, a programme for rural general practice nurses is offered jointly by the Department of Clinical Nursing and the Department of General Practice, both situated with the School of Medicine at The University of Adelaide.

Entrepreneurial skills

Nurses have good communication and teamwork skills; they are generally deficient in management and other business and entrepreneurial skills. A FPN (reported as a case study in Chapter Five) setting up a private practice to a rural community needed skills in entrepreneurship, business management and marketing. As Goodyear comments, education in the traditional nursing programmes does not encompass these concepts or skills. If nurses are to make an impact on the future of healthcare, preparation in these skills is vital.

Marketing involves developing a good service and raising its profile so that it becomes visible to those with the desire and power to purchase it. It can take many forms; indeed it is most effective when it does so. The case study of good practice in health professions education described in Chapter Six is very successful in marketing what it has to offer. CCPH promote best practice by teaching, research, mounting conferences and by provision of a quarterly newsletter which flags case studies of good practice as 'Models that Work'. They also have a regular item showcasing the activities and views of leaders. Ramely (1999) is showcased in her position as President of the University of Vermont. She is reported as having a passion for the public purpose of higher education. In her inaugural speech she commented:

> We must prepare our students to exercise their responsibilities as citizens. Furthermore, we must demonstrate by our own conduct the civic responsibility that we must exercise as a community of scholars. Increasingly, we are challenged to draw on our intellectual resources to understand and address the problems of contemporary society and to strengthen our role of 'university citizen'. Through public service and civic involvement, we also provide our students with excellent learning opportunities.

Nationally and internationally, throughout the last decade, nursing and health organisations have exhorted nurses to show leadership skills, yet too often failed to recognise that leadership involves teamwork, negotiation and other management of change skills. Generally, nurses have been poorly prepared in these skills (Spitzer, 1998):

> The crisis that is evident in nursing today caused both by lack of role definition and absence of strong leadership, is a clear sign that we did not read the writing on the wall . . . nursing is being challenged by the new paradigm of the changing healthcare system but with little preparation as to how to cope.

Advanced practice nurses cannot afford to be inadequately prepared in leadership and management of change skills. Not only will they fail to make the best contribution possible to patient service and organisational effectiveness and efficiency, but their contribution will also remain invisible.

Leadership skills

The call for leadership is loud and it is international. In the US, The Pew Commission (1995) a 'blue ribbon panel of health care leaders' recommended that nurses:

- practice leadership
- work in interdisciplinary teams
- use information technology effectively and appropriately.

In the US, CCPH responded to the challenge of the Pew Commission by developing interdisciplinary service–learning for health professionals (*see* Chapter Six). CCPH is a new, government-supported national initiative; it therefore stands a good chance of being successful. Difficulties in changing the attitudes and practices of nurse educators working in traditional institutions persist however, and have been commented on earlier. The RCN Futures Report (1998) describes nurse educators as still being seen as out of touch with clinical nursing and the example of professors of medicine who retain clinical responsibilities: 'was often cited as a way forward for the academic nurse.'

In their defence, educators are reported as arguing that workloads in the Departments of Nursing often prohibited other activities, and also that part of the problem was that practice involvement was not seen as a priority area for nurses in academic settings. This was also an issue for the educator described in Chapter Nine who failed to get faculty support for a new service-led interdisciplinary course. There are now, however, signs that things may start to get easier. As the CCPH initiative expands in the US, attitudes and practices will change. In Europe international collaboration in university/service collaborative healthcare provision is growing. De Maeseneer and Derese (1998) report on university and community service partnerships in primary care education in a number of European countries. Collaboration in service-led curriculum development in Australia (Adelaide) was commented on earlier in the chapter.

So what advice do those who are involved in service-led education offer? The lessons provided by CCPH (US) are:

- **To develop a faculty champion**. Leadership plays an important role in supporting service–learning efforts. The grant funding of the programme supported a health sciences campus service–learning co-ordinator. This faculty member served as the support for other faculty who wanted to implement service–learning but lacked the knowledge of the community, or felt that they did not have the time to commit to developing community placement

- **To tie the development into the regular programme of faculty development** to both change the institutional context and build ownership of the changes.
- **To find new ways of rewarding educators for their efforts and recognise innovation in teaching practice as a valid professional activity for career advancement** (as opposed to a single reliance on publications record, which may only advance the individual concerned).

Changes in both health and education policy in the UK are requiring professional education to be more useful to the community for which it is meant to serve, and clinical leadership in nursing is to be made easier and be rewarded. The UK Strategy for Nursing document (DoH, 1999) aims to promote movement into and upwards through the profession. Launching it the Prime Minister said (Blair, 1999):

> *Nurses, midwives and health visitors are often constrained by structures that limit development and innovation.*

With regard to advanced practice the goal is to reward nurses who stay in, and lead, clinical practice. Salaries of up to £40 000 (30% more than the current cap) are promised for nurse consultants, who are seen as numbering thousands *'within a few years'*. It is envisaged that these expert practitioners will spend at least half their time in clinical practice (patient contact), provide expert, evidence-based practice, and leadership, mentorship and consultancy to other nurses and health workers.

Nurses in the UK are ready to seize the opportunity. The RCN and the Kings Fund Institute (of Health Policy) have been researching and developing leadership education for nurses for a number of years. A leading researcher/educator is Malby (1997) who provides a profile for the nurse leader for the millennium. She will be:

- a strategist; able to develop and implement strategy
- an environmentalist; able to adapt the organisation to a changing environment, to look at ways to make the organisation effective locally, and at ways of managing information
- a politically aware operator; able to work with national and local priorities and to use political awareness to the benefit of the organisation
- a confident leader; able to contribute fully to board-level working, and to the professional development of nursing, and able to lead beyond hierarchy in complex organisations.

The leader:

- has well-developed process/consultancy skills
- has a sense of purpose
- is self-aware and able to recognise and maximise personal impact
- is comfortable with themselves and able to express themselves through their work.

These characteristics are helpful for nurse education, and for recruitment to leadership positions in nursing. The dilemma seems to be whether the profession should focus its efforts on developing the leadership skills of all post-basic nurses (nursing policy documents seem to imply this), or whether they should concentrate their efforts on developing an elite corps of nursing leaders.

Commenting on the crisis in nursing leadership (poor, reactive, slow, politically naïve) Evers (1997) suggests that:

> . . . our efforts be concentrated on an elite group of talented youngsters for clinical leadership roles in nursing. The aim is to prepare students for clinical and managerial nursing leadership roles in a healthcare system where the focus is on decentralization and managed care. The aim is to prepare students for research-based practice in a healthcare system where the focus is on quality service, i.e. on effective and efficient patient care. The aim is also to develop a scientific nursing knowledge base in a healthcare system where the focus is on handling the increasing demand for nursing-care functions. The last aim is the only legitimate reason for graduate university education at masters and doctoral level.

Leadership in clinical practice is the goal of the Doctoral Nursing (DN) programme of the University of Adelaide which sees its function as preparing clinical nurse graduates who are able to act effectively in a leadership role (Pearson *et al.*, 1997). In developing the DN programme, educators saw the need for preparation at the highest level, which would be different to PhD preparation:

> There is growing evidence supporting the usefulness of this approach [PhD] in preparing researchers and academics; but industry and the professions argue that the PhD is not serving them well in preparing either team players who can engage in research from a variety of paradigmatic positions, or professional leaders who can advance the theory and practice of nursing's contribution to societal health and well-being . . . Nurses who are able to see that healthcare should be placed

within the bigger picture of a world characterised by scarce resources, complex social problems and an ageing population are better placed to influence decisions positively and control the changes.

The University of Adelaide DN programme requires students to build a portfolio of excellence in which evidence of leading and sustaining change in an interdisciplinary healthcare context is provided.

Service-linked leadership preparation of practitioners is more educationally sound than when studied in the abstract. The success of School of Nursing programmes at McMaster University (Canada) are also testament to this. For their Leadership Training for Development programme, interdisciplinary teams of faculty and students participate in educational and service exchange programmes that both develop curricula skills and address local health needs. Smith *et al.* (1992) describe a leadership skills' programme in which women's health was the lead issue. Ten interdisciplinary teams from health sciences institutions worldwide participated in an education project. Project objectives included:

- increasing participants' awareness of women's health issues globally
- increasing participants' abilities as future decision makers in health-care
- developing action-orientated, sustainable and local strategies for health in their home setting.

Following leadership education and a three-week country exchange visit students further designed, implemented and evaluated local strategies addressing primary healthcare. They did this in partnership with the community. This trend of professional/citizen collaboration is one which is increasing as citizens become more informed about healthcare choices. A major source of information is the Internet. It is estimated that 250 million people will have Internet access in the year 2000, and use is growing rapidly (Samli *et al.*, 1997). It is predicted that people will become more informed about, and demanding of, health practice (Warner *et al.*, 1998):

. . . As a communication channel, benefits for the consumer in relation to healthcare include extended search and comparison of interventions and treatment options, with high information content and feedback from others.

Describing the future these authors go on to predict that:

Within healthcare itself, computers and telecommunications will make it possible to tie all parts of the healthcare system together. The implications of improving co-ordination and communication through these tools have hardly been explored: routine data systems will greatly expand the possibilities of research, and computer-based feedback systems will revolutionise quality assurance.

Information technology skills

Nurses have not yet embraced information technology. In addition to entrepreneurial, marketing and leadership skills, nurses need to improve their information technology skills. They need to become fully computer literate and to design their own projects of excellence, rather than just entering data for others. Knowledge about and use of technology is a fundamental tool of enfranchisement in the new century. The concern for nurses (most of whom are women) is that women have been slow to embrace the information society: and, when they have, the evidence is that the gender segregation that affected women in traditional work is being repeated; men design the projects, women punch in the data (Houdart-Blazy, 1996).

A large amount of technophobia still exists amongst nurses. The RCN Futures Project (1998) reported that:

While some nurses had embraced the potential of information technology with enthusiasm, most viewed it with scepticism if not fear. There was widespread misunderstanding about the relevance of computers to nursing practice, perhaps underscored by the perception that computers had thus far been primarily introduced for management and cost-control purposes rather than direct aids to better patient care. Participants consistently reported fears about the technological age, although many nurses reported owning their own computers. The skill gap between what most nurses know about IT and the advances in its use was often a cause for concern.

Use of the information society is both the main challenge and opportunity facing nurses today. The potential exists for nurses to initiate, develop and showcase change in practice. Two initiatives illustrating this are described briefly below.

PC networking for remote northern health centres is a community health nurse-initiated and run information technology service to a remote area of Canada, Prince Albert in Saskatchewan (Huang *et al.*, 1994). The Prince Albert Grand Council (PAGC) consists of 12 member

First Nations, and 23 commnunities. Together they comprise 40% of the Province of Saskatchewan. Within the Grand Council there are five tribal groups; Plains Cree, Swampy Cree, Woodland Cree, Dene and Dakota. Each group is described as having distinct traditions, culture and language. Since 1992 the PAGC has taken control of services, including health promotion, mental health, community health development, environmental health, addictions, research and epidemiology. PAGC provide community nursing supervision to staff at health centres by a simple personalised computer (PC) network. It has two components:

- central co-ordination and information support
- local working stations supported by on-site and remote training.

The goal is to streamline the health centre administration system, enhance the centre's ability to access the latest public health and medical information, and strengthen the First Nation's management capacities. The project team describe how they went about their task, emphasising the need to be realistic and flexible:

> During the planning stage the Information Superhighway was a very hot topic. However we realized that we are working to build a basic information highway, not a super-highway. We also realized that not everyone comes onto the road with the same driving skills. We tried to use the simplest information technology available to meet our iden-tified needs. In a northern setting, the telephone system provides the least expensive, in most instances the only way to do computer networking. Hooking our network with Health Canada's Bulletin Board Service (BBS) gives us free access to the latest public health information while connect-ing us with other Canadian health professionals.

Low-cost, easy-access, socially inclusive technologies were also the subject of a nurse led European research project; **Telematics for Health** (Gott, 1995). The study was commissioned because of a growing concern in Europe (but universally applicable) that medical technology has not been supporting the 'Health for All' principles of social justice and equitable access to health services (WHO, 1978).

High-tech care (medical, hospital) has created a dramatic rise in healthcare expenditure worldwide, yet the pay off has been slight (Dutton, 1988; Konner, 1993). Rising demand for healthcare has forced countries to examine options for changing systems of service delivery. Telemedicine is one of the main options advocated (Gott, 1995):

> **Telemedicine** *is the investigation, monitoring and management of patients and the education of patients and staff using systems which allow ready access to expert advice, no matter where the patient is located.*

There is a place for the growth of telemedicine in healthcare, but not the hegemonically dominant place that it now occupies. Health is about more than physiological functioning. It is about the welfare and quality of life of whole people in whole communities. The project established a case for investing in telehealth (Gott, 1995):

> **Telehealth** *is the promotion and facilitation of health and well-being with individuals and communities by use of telematic services.*

Case studies of good practice in telehealth have been described in Europe, the US and Canada. All used simple, accessible, low-cost technologies. They included:

- remote (modem) domiciliary foetal monitoring of high-risk pregnant women
- a CD-ROM-based information system for the disabled
- an electronic Bulletin Board System (BBS) for youth anti-drug education
- personal alarms to support independent living and early hospital discharge of vulnerable patients (some premature babies and post-surgery 'seniors')
- videotelephone support for independent living and improvement of mental health
- technologies to support public participation in decision making (electronic voting on government health policies).

The author concludes:

> *. . . the social technologies (television, telephone, videophone) have an important role to play in promoting the health and well-being of European citizens. To use these most effectively, however, it is necessary to revalue, and listen to, all citizens of Europe (including the young, disabled and elderly). It is also necessary to focus on the settings where most of life is lived: the home and the community.*

Revaluing society has been a theme much in evidence at the turn of the millennium. A marker has been provided against which people can take stock of achievements and failures. A major problem with the 20th century was its phallocentric western bias. New times call for new approaches.

Changing health policy: the female future

A gender shift is evident in society, as people increasingly reject the masculine value system that dominated public policy and public life throughout the previous century. Female values are gaining public recognition. Feminine values are holistic and inclusive, rather than individual and exclusive (male). They offer the potential for a different kind of healthcare that focuses on the long- rather than the short-term, and the broad, rather than the narrow gaze. Thinking about the social future Giddens (1996) cites the value of incorporating the female perspective into welfare planning and advocates a new social contract between men and women as the key to positive welfare:

> *Women across the world now stake a claim for forms of autonomy previously denied or unavailable to them. Such a claim plainly has a strong emancipatory element, in so far as a struggle is involved to achieve equal economic and political rights with men. At the same time, however, that claim to autonomy intrudes deeply into the domain of life politics, for it raises issues to do with the very domain of what it is to be a woman, and therefore a man, in detraditionalizing societies and cultures. Few things can be more significant worldwide than the possibility of a new social contract between women and men . . .*

Giddens and other leading thinkers are now calling for re-appraisal of the direction in which societies are headed, and making a plea for a return to (female, nursing) human scale and human values. In her exploration of the contribution of feminism to modern society Coward (1999) recognises that the world of work is rapidly changing and the skills that are valued now are flexibility and 'female' communication skills.

Fisher (1999) theorises that the way women think and work is the way society needs to develop in the future. In forming her thesis about how the female mind has evolved, and is 'wired' differently to the male mind, Fisher reviewed evidence from the fields of psychology, sociology, medicine and economics and concluded that women's ability to multitask, work in teams, build consensus and weigh options are the qualities that will be vital for working in the third millennium.

It seems that the ideological tide might be turning in nurses' favour. But they are not quite ready to capitalise on it. Internationally and nationally, professional nursing organisations need to focus their attention on preparing nurses for leadership in healthcare. This is different to leadership in nursing. Of course we need both, but have generally only recognised the need for the latter. The nurses in the RCN Futures project recognised the distinction:

> Views on leadership were polarised between those who perceived a lack of nursing leaders ('the voice of nursing is not being heard in the corridors of power') and those who saw leadership being invested at clinical level (described as 'we need to recognise and use the leadership in each of us').

Given the opportunity to influence policy, nurses will take it. Chambers (Chapter Three) describes how nurse practitioners in her study sought out opportunities. Two had gained a management role within the PHC practice; one managing the two practice nurses and participating fully in practice management meetings with the partners and the practice manager, the other co-ordinating all nursing activity across practice nursing, district nursing and health visiting. Another nurse practitioner was reported as being the nurse representative on the local (service commissioning) subcommittee for the PGC to which the practice belongs. She also had taken on responsibilities for developing and maintaining good relations with the community nurses in the locality.

Chambers comments that these nurses were demonstrating an eagerness and assertiveness to participate in decision making about primary care issues far beyond the concerns of the practice nurse treatment room, whilst still retaining and developing their clinical expertise. It appears that 'triggers' were twofold: the 'permission' given by their extended role, but also the experience of higher level education courses with exposure to the power politics inherent in nursing and medicine.

The experience of the nurses in the Derbyshire project suggests that going on the higher level courses teaches not only advanced clinical expertise, but also a greater assertiveness which allows nurses to take their place alongside, rather than as assistants to, family doctors.

Goodyear (Chapter Five) also links higher education with greater assertiveness. She describes nurses who have had to change their practice because of limitations imposed by managed care, but who have found different ways to continue to practice and even to grow. By sharing their stories these nurses provide valuable case material for managers, educationalists and others facing change.

Articulate, informed nurses need to be involved in all levels of health service decision making. Part of their role will be to educate other health service decision makers about the value of nursing. That should start with a challenge to the stereotypical view of a 'nurse'; held by some within, as well as outside of, the healthcare profession. Salvage (1999) argues that many people are unaware of the real nature of nursing work and especially of the skills and knowledge required to do it well. Challenging the stereotype of the nurse at the bedside (and the doctors side!) she points out:

> *We have nurses as expert clinicians, counsellors, managers, teachers, researchers, professors, policy-makers, civil servants, trade union leaders, even magazine editors.*

A better understanding of the range encompassed by nursing will lead to a better understanding of the contribution nursing can make to the health and well-being of society. This is particularly urgent at this time as, worldwide, governments are seeking to limit health service budgets and exploring 'skill mix' forms of service provision. Spitzer (1998) argues:

> *Without a clear understanding of nursing's relative contribution and in need of choosing the most efficient and cost-contained workforce, provider organizations . . . are not necessarily finding nurses to be the best care solution in the radically changing healthcare system. The hard data on the increasing numbers of nursing positions being absorbed, and the harsh competition among nurse and various allied health professionals are indications of the acuity of the problem.*

Spitzer is referring to the situation in the US, but the problem is international. Referring to the opportunities for nursing outlined in a UK government policy document (DoH, 1997) an editorial in *Health Visitor* (1998) points out:

> *Yes, the door is open, but without the establishment of some form of community nursing network to support nurses on primary care groups they will have to be superhuman to get their voices heard . . .it is ironic that this long-term vision for a better health service comes at a time when health service managers are being forced to take short-term decisions which are affecting hundreds of community nursing jobs. Unless the*

> *government acts now and gives guidance to health service managers that the current budget restraints must not lead to more community nursing cuts, its long-term vision for the NHS will be scuppered by a distinct lack of community practitioners able to sit on primary care groups.*

The intention to create new nurse consultant posts in the UK has been referred to earlier. Whilst the profession has cautiously welcomed the plan, it remains sceptical about the number of posts that will be created, and therefore the influence these nurses will have.

Gough (1999) argues that it is in the governments' interest to ensure that more (rather than few) nurse consultant posts are created, in order to tackle recruitment and retention problems:

> *If nurses see the career path as a pyramid with very steep sides and only a few nurse consultants at the top, the government will lose nurses for ever.*

As is often the case, there is no new money to implement the reforms discussed above. Nurses have been down this road before, and are right to be cautious of protestations of admiration. The difference between this and previous nursing strategy documents, however, is that this one gives a good indication of knowing what nursing is, and can be. Commenting on the strategy document Salvage (1999) said:

> *It goes further than the usual rhetoric; it recognises that nurses can do more than has previously been recognised, and that they can be cost-effective health workers. It's weak and disappointing on leadership and processes though . . . nurses have always found gaps in the system where they can practice in different ways . . . will the new strategy facilitate this? . . . I don't know.*

On balance it could be argued that the signs are favourable. The value of advanced practice nurses as flexible, efficient, cost-effective health practitioners is one which is increasingly being recognised, across the world. In Australia this has resulted in quite speedy legislation to recognise and protect their practice. Within three years of the New South Wales Nurse Practitioner trials, the enabling legislation was passed by both houses of parliament. In 1999, nurse practitioners in South Australia gained clinical, prescribing and admitting privileges. These rights are also enjoyed by some US nurses (*see* Chapter Nine). The UK will not be able to ignore this policy trend. In 1998 the UKCC commissioned a healthcare futures report (Warner *et al.*, 1998). It predicts three alternative scenarios:

- muddling through; economic stringency and no clear leadership of health policy
- continuation of current policies, based on economic strength and consumer choice
- expansion of the free market and individual choice in healthcare; reduction in NHS expenditure.

In all three scenarios, growth of nursing at the 'top end' (advanced practice) is predicted, together with growth in employment of autonomous nurses with increased technical skills, prescribing and admitting rights. Growth in provision of nurse-led services is also foreseen.

Conclusion: advancing nursing and healthcare practice

Nurses are an underused healthcare asset. However, their value is now being universally recognised by governments anxious to achieve cost-effective and skill-efficient health service provision for the future. Nurses are worth investing in. Given appropriate education, legislation and development opportunities, nurses will deliver innovative, context-sensitive, evidence-based health promotion and illness care services.

The case studies of good practice and the supportive evidence provided in this book indicate that nurses are ready to face the future. They are cautious about it, and rightly so. The 20th century was not generous to them, either as nurses or as women. Significant gains have been made, however. Nursing gains include:

- education at the highest level
- expansion of clinical practice
- acceptance as equals in the healthcare team
- representation in healthcare decision-making groups
- collaboration with (often underserved) citizens and communities to reduce inequalities in access to healthcare.

When reviewing change, too often the outcomes are celebrated, and the processes by which they were achieved are forgotten. The case studies and related discussion contained in this book provide detailed material about how some nurses have advanced their professional practice and the opportunities and obstacles they have faced on the way. Their stories are a gift to the profession as it begins to map its way into a promising but uncertain future.

References

Adebajo CF (1998) The potential role of nursing and midwifery personnel in public health. *Nursing/Midwifery Discussion Paper No 2.* World Health Organisation, Geneva.

Blair T (1999) Comments reported by D Brindle and M White: new deal for nurses. *The Guardian* 9 July: 1.

Coward R (1999) *Sacred Cows: Is Feminism Relevant to the New Millennium?* Harper Collins, New York.

De Maeseneer J and Derese A (1998) Meeting priority health goals: a joint contribution of health professionals and academic institutions. *Changing Medical Education and Medical Practice* **13**.

DoH (1997) *The New NHS.* Department of Health, London.

DoH (1999) *Making a Difference. Strengthening the Nursing, Midwifery and Health Visiting Contribution to Health and Healthcare.* Department of Health, London.

Dutton DB (1988) *Worse than the Disease. Pitfalls of Medical Progress.* Cambridge University Press, Cambridge.

Editorial (1998) *Health Visitor* **71**(1): 3.

Evers GCM (1997) The future role of nursing and nurses in the European Union. *European Nurse* **2**(3): 171–9.

Fisher H (1999) *The First Sex: The Natural Talents of Women and How They are Changing the World.* Random House, New York.

Giddens A (1996) Affluence, poverty and the idea of a post scarcity society. In: LCH de Alcantara *Social Futures, Global Visions.* Blackwell Publishers, Oxford.

Gott M (1995) *Telematics for Health. The role of telehealth and telemedicine in homes and communities.* Radcliffe Medical Press, Oxford.

Gough P (1999) In: D Payne Nice work if you can get it. *Nursing Times* **95**(29): 12.

Heathrow Debate (1994) *The Challenges for Nursing and Midwifery in the 21st Century.* Department of Health, London.

Hine D (1999) For the good that it will do: issues confronting healthcare in the UK. *Journal of the Royal Society of Medicine* **92**: 332–8.

Houdart-Blazy (1996) Introduction: the information society . . . a challenge for women. *Women of Europe Dossier* **44**. European Commission, Brussels.

Huang J, Merasty J and Safnuk T (1994) *PC Networking For Remote Northern Health Centres.* Information Technology in Community Health Conference, 30 October–2 November, Victoria, Canada: 1–11.

Konner M (1993) *The Trouble With Medicine.* BBC Books, London.

Malby R (1997) Developing the future leaders of nursing in the UK. *European Nurse* **2**(1): 27–35.

Pearson A, Borbasi S and Gott M (1997) Doctoral education in nursing for practitioner knowledge and for academic knowledge: the University of Adelaide, Australia. *Image: Journal of Nursing Scholarship* **29**(4): 365–8.

Ramely R (1999) Showcasing leaders. *Partnership Matters Newsletter* **2**(1). University of California, San Francisco.

RCN (1998) *Imagining The Future. Nursing in The New Millennium.* Royal College of Nursing, London.

RSM (1998) Telemedicine Forum. 30th June. Royal Society of Medicine, London.

Salvage J (1999) *Carry On, Nurse.* NHS 50th Anniversary Lecture Series. National Health Service Executive, Leeds.

Samli AL, Willis JR and Herbig G (1997) The information superhighway goes international. *The Journal of Marketing Management* **26**: 51–8.

Seifer S (1997) *Overcoming a Century of Town-Gown Relations: Redefining Relationships Between Communities and Academic Health Centers. Expanding Boundaries: Service and Learning.* Corporation for National Service, Washington.

Smith SE, Carpio B and Sanderson-Godlewski D (1992) *Women and health: leadership training for development.* Proceedings of the International Colloquium on Primary Healthcare, Montreal, 21–23 May.

Spitzer A (1998) Nursing in the healthcare system of the postmodern world: crossroads, paradoxes and complexity. *Journal of Advanced Nursing* **28**(1): 164–71.

Warner M, Longley M, Gould E and Picek A (1998) *Healthcare Futures 2010.* United Kingdom Central Council for Nursing, Midwifery and Health Visiting, London.

WHO (1978, and subsequent) *Alma Ata Declaration* (on Health For All). WHO Regional Office for Europe, Copenhagen.

Index